*Constellations* is a beautiful gift to communities of freedom-minded people, offering a glimpse into many worlds of possibility. Across the many authors and experiences represented, deeply resonating themes of nurturing love and fierce resilience intertwine in a tapestry of hope.

—Kai Cheng Thom, author of *Falling Back in Love
with Being Human*

With rare candor and rigorous insight, Cindy Barukh Milstein's anthologies offer the conversations we need to sustain the communal possibility of anarchist, feminist, and queer world-making in the ruins of everyday brutality.

—Mattilda Bernstein Sycamore, author of *Touching the Art*

An antidote to the commodification of care, *Constellations* brings together a multiplicity of voices on the subject, in an approach that makes visible the intentionality and diversity of care practices.

—Sundus Abdul Hadi, author of *Take Care of Your Self:
The Art and Cultures of Care and Liberation*

*Constellations of Care* brings together all kinds of veterans of liberatory experiments in comradeship and kin-making, providing valuable insight into obstacles and defeats as well as tales of abundant love saplings, spores, and cuttings for everyone to propagate and grow.

—Sophie Lewis, author of *Abolish the Family:
A Manifesto for Care and Liberation*

T0279685

# CONSTELLATIONS OF CARE

## ANARCHA-FEMINISM IN PRACTICE

CON

LAT

OF C

STEL

IONS

CARE

## ANARCHA-FEMINISM IN PRACTICE

*Edited by Cindy Barukh Milstein*

PLUTO PRESS

First published 2024 by Pluto Press
New Wing, Somerset House, Strand, London WC2R 1LA
and Pluto Press, Inc.
1930 Village Center Circle, 3-834, Las Vegas, NV 89134

www.plutobooks.com

British Library Cataloguing in Publication Data
A catalogue record for this book is available from the British Library

ISBN 978 0 7453 4995 4        Paperback
ISBN 978 0 7453 4997 8        PDF
ISBN 978 0 7453 4996 1        EPUB

Cover design by Crisis
Interior design by Geraldine Hendler
All author royalties go to various anarcha-feminist initiatives.

This book is printed on paper suitable for recycling and made from fully managed
and sustained forest sources. Logging, pulping and manufacturing processes are
expected to conform to the environmental standards of the country of origin.

Printed in the United Kingdom

To you, all of you,
who embody anarcha-feminism every day.
Who tend unceasingly to life.
Who too often are unseen.
Without you, the ground would crumble
and the stars would fall.

# CONTENTS

# PROLOGUE: CONSTELLATIONS OF CARE

/

CINDY BARUKH MILSTEIN

If we set our aims on destroying hierarchies, ... [we should] devise social relations that no longer reproduce that world. Our actions right now prefigure the world we want, and will help end the world that tries to contain us. We can taste the old world's death in our relations that extricate its logic and control.

—Scott Branson, "For a Tranarchist Feminism," 2023

There is an element here that is not explicit but that is fundamental: practice. ... We are not talking about something that could be, we are talking about something that we are already doing. ... Our rebellion is our "NO" to the system. Our resistance is our "YES" to something else being possible.

—Sub Galeano, "The Method, the Bibliography, and a Drone," 2015

Daily, hourly, for over sixty-seven days while struggling—and failing—to write this prologue, I've been witnessing—or rather, feeling—the rubble. The bodies. The genocide. The system that our ancestors said "NO" to again and again for millennia across so many geographies. The system that we're now watching in real time via images from Palestinians on the ground in Gaza.

Across an aching world, we add our "NO," with our feet and our solidarity, yet it falls silently on the ears of those who only hear the siren call of hierarchy and control.

So of course words fail me. Fail us.

As one poignant essay observed recently, we are experiencing "grief beyond language."[1] Which is another way of saying that we're experiencing rage beyond language, bundled in a "pain and sadness so big that they no longer fit in the heart of a few," as the Zapatistas observed in a communiqué on January 1, 1994, but instead demand a shared, collective heart.[2]

We need, as we always have, the "YES" of our practices: constellations of care, where each and every one of our still-beating hearts, in concert, rebelliously speaks louder than words, forming unmistakable patterns of different cosmologies, different worlds, life against their death machine.

This happens, as it always has and likely always will, within an imperfect universe, where we're guided by billions of points of our own self-generated light—all the resistance that came before us and is shining brightly now—even as those who seek dominion strive to extinguish our luminosity.

I'm reminded here of a Shabbat evening not so long ago, in the first year of another ongoing catastrophe, COVID-19. A small group of us queer+trans Jews circled up in a narrow Pittsburgh backyard, sandwiched between row houses and barking dogs, to share and sing songs of joy, sorrow, and rebellion for hours. As our bodies increasingly coregulated, brought into sacred connection in opposition to the cruel isolation of societal abandonment, I turned my face upward,

---

1. Nicki Kattoura and Nada Abuasi, "Grief beyond Language," Institute for Palestine Studies, October 27, 2023, https://palestine-studies.org/en/node/1654517.

2. Quoted in Dylan Elderidge Fitzwater, *Autonomy Is in Our Hearts: Zapatista Autonomous Government through the Lens of the Tzotzil Language* (Oakland, CA: PM Press, 2019), 31.

bedazzled by the ancient stars, and took in a breath of the world as it should be. Then I saw antisemitic billionaire Elon Musk's Starlink satellites begin their crawl from one horizon of the night sky, with an assured hubris, until they stretched fully across it. "NO," I screamed, shattering our a cappella harmony, and all eyes looked above. We paused, honoring the loss of the firmament and so much else to capitalism and colonialism, patriarchy and fascism, and then looked back into each other's eyes, in the time-space we were reclaiming, beyond their thefts, and raised our voices in melodic defiance again.

I'm reminded of how, soon after the start of this latest Nakba chapter, another group of rad Jews in another city, Asheville, leaned into our centuries-old technologies of grief practices, inseparable from our histories of ungovernable political practices. We organized and held time-space for a Mourner's Kaddish, which as many stories have it, became linked to loss and mourning in response to the Crusades' murderous brutality toward Jewish communities in the thirteenth century. Our "Jews against genocide" public Mourner's Kaddish, outdoors by a well-used river trail, gathered well over two hundred people of various ethnicities, ages, genders, and faiths (or not) to join in creating an expansive DIY altar in solidarity with Palestinians and sharing in the fullness of raw emotions. We knew that we couldn't stop the bombing— for as anarchists, we recognize that would entail a seismic shift in the overarching social order—but we assuredly understood, as anarcha-feminists, that it is well within our power to forge social relations that point beyond nation-states.

So we did what states don't want us to do and frequently

try to stymie, such as in Gaza: collectively mourn, honor, and remember our dead. By not skipping over our trauma and grief, by extending empathy to each other and "consoling the dead lest [we] give up on the cause of living," by "beckon[ing] forth a humanism that has to be constructed," we sustain, as Nadia Bou Ali asserts in a contemporary piece, "the very question of what it means to live, to be alive," in all the ways that Christo-fascism and white supremacy unceasingly attempt to crush.[3] Indeed, such do-it-ourselves rituals of resistance are crucial to why people fight so hard for the living. We depicted that sensibility in an enormous banner framing our Kaddish altar. It read "Never again means never again for any people." Perhaps more to the point, we'd decided to paint luscious olives and a juicy pomegranate on either side of these words, rather than nationalistic or statist images and their flags, to symbolize lengthy, lived practices of interwovenness beyond borders—the trees of life that we, ourselves, plant from the countless seeds of "YES."

It shouldn't take a genocide to "beckon forth" our better selves and the preciousness of life. Yet whether we like it or not—and I abhor it—we are face-to-face with a genocidal, nay, ecocidal period of (in)human history. And potentialities for other pathways don't arise from theories removed from the here-and-nowness of this everyday devastation, nor do lives worth living. They emerge from the humus we cultivate, as in the two examples above.

It's a big reason that I return, time and again, to the Zapatistas. They've demonstrated their theory not through

_____

3. Nadia Bou Ali, "Ugly Enjoyment," *Parapraxis*, accessed December 12, 2023, https://parapraxismagazine.com/articles/ugly-enjoyment.

the halls of academia or armchairs of intellectuals—those who have everything to gain from maintaining the deadening status quo—but instead via their actual practices and lived experiences of them, relayed through the wit and wisdom of storytelling, a tradition that harks back to the dawn of human language. For over three decades now, when the Zapatistas bump up against new hierarchies or those they hadn't fully noticed before, both outside and within their own autonomous communities, they've also embellished on those tales—at once poetry and promise—to humbly detail needed refinements to their practices.

This ability to journey side by side with each other toward liberatory vistas we can barely yet imagine but enact deeply in our daily relations, constructively amending our circuitous course as we go, and generously swapping stories and sustenance along the way around the warmth of rebel campfires, real and metaphoric, has the quality of what might be called *anarcha-feminism*. This anthology doesn't try to pin down a precise definition because that would limit possibilities and destinations. It would turn anarcha-feminism into a static, passive term, or a hollow phrase on a dos-and-don'ts list posted on the walls of a social center. In contrast, the contributors to this collection make use of their anarcha-feminism, whether they explicitly use that self-descriptor or not, and for sure in ways that *queer* and *trans*form it, as a verb. They carry it as an ethical compass that perpetually guides how we, ourselves, routinely take "positive" direct actions, "wherein our actions directly open up room for blissful other possible worlds—not merely in our hearts, but in our actual lives."[4]

So this book asks you, its readers, to gather for a story share about "anarcha-feminism in practice"—stories that together, like stars of various shapes, sizes, and brilliance, converge into discernible celestial patterns, "constellations of care" that bring the otherworldly dreams of this praxis down to earth—this imperiled earth. The pieces in this volume implicitly speak honest, dignified truths *against* top-down power by exploring how we act to prefiguratively *disperse* power from below. Such practices can only be "read" through their engendering and doing, experiencing and feeling, tinkering with and reveling in, commoning and sharing. They don't vie for fame or profit, power or control, but rather continually embody forms of life and care, love and solidarity, always against the grain of what wants to destroy all of that, all of us, along with the whole of our ecosystem.

Certainly, the aspirations of anarchism have always, at their core, revolved around what could be understood as "feminist" ethics—self-determination and bodily autonomy, voluntaristic and consensual association as well as responsibility, egalitarian social relations and relationship building, mutual aid and social solidarity, and loving freely as well as queerly, to mention a few. Moreover, the bulk of what we anarchists have actually done in practice, and still do, imperfectly and yet beautifully, falls under the banner of self-organized collective care, freely gifted—or again, what could be seen as feminist ethics, in which we have one another's backs and know that others have ours. We shouldn't have to,

---

4. Cindy Barukh Milstein, *Try Anarchism for Life: The Beauty of Our Circle* (Strangers in a Tangled Wilderness, 2022), 69.

in short, add *feminism*; it should be self-evident in the word *anarchism*. Likewise, the aspirations of feminism should be indistinguishable from an anarchist ethics, toward the abolition of gender as a category that oppresses, assaults, or otherwise does violence to the wholeness of who we all could be, freed from the dominance of cisheteronormativity and prevalence of misogyny.

Yet for a host of reasons—ranging from toxic "male" behaviors and patriarchal power structures within our own anarchist circles, to liberalism, racism, classism, and transphobia, among others, busily trying to eviscerate the *radical* from feminist circles—the aspirations and practices of communal care have long been devalued, demeaned, or destroyed, or made invisible. And not merely by individuals— although it is indeed done frequently by individuals—but systemically. To borrow from the Zapatistas again, "We must not forget that when the system has to choose a gender, it chooses to be masculine, male, man, macho—even when it is administered by a woman."[5]

If we're serious about fundamentally, nay, radically (as in "getting to the roots") transforming this world, including in joyfully militant and riotously joyful ways, we must be serious about simultaneously transforming ourselves. Anarcha-feminists have long articulated this notion. We've underscored too, in words and deeds, that there's no binary between social relations and social organization, or what's been called "the personal" and "the political." Instead, there's a developmental logic, nurtured through the ways we act as

---

5. Sub Galeano, "Halves, Thirds, Fourths," in *Critical Thought in the Face of the Capitalist Hydra I*, by Sixth Commission of the EZLN (Durham, NC: PaperBoat Press, 2016), 197.

if we were already free people in a free society, allowing us to "taste" nonhierarchical worlds coming to life.

Now, in the dumpster fire of the nonstop disasters we confront as a species, there's no ignoring what feministic anarchists—these days, thankfully, inseparable from or another way of describing queer, trans, and gender-nonconforming anarchists—have been arguing all along: "We are all we have." No one, as they say, is coming to rescue us, nor as anarchists did we ever think they would. So we must also be, passionately, abidingly, and with fierce love, "all we need" and desire. Whether one is an anarchist or not, the contemporary turn of geopolitical events—from the global phenomena of pandemics, fascistic regimes, and collapsing infrastructure for any sort of social well-being, to capitalist-fueled climate catastrophes and displacement, to occupations spiraling into genocides—has compelled a shift toward prioritizing do-it-ourselves forms of taking good care of each other. Suddenly, the many anarcha-feministic practices that previously felt like "nothing" when people didn't take the time or care to notice them—or worse, didn't take the time or care to engage in those practices themselves—now feel like, and indeed are, everything.

Or as Nicole Rose of Solidarity Apothecary eloquently puts it in her contribution,

> Care is a radical act, and one of our biggest weapons. Collective care points beyond all the structures we fight against while simultaneously already embodying the alternatives we fight and yearn for. Yet for too long, the centrality of care to life itself has been downplayed

or erased, including within anarchist circles. Anarcha-feminists have challenged the invisibilization of care, even as they've typically been the ones to engage in the myriad types of "care work" that form the backbone of anarchist infrastructure, and are essential to everything that anarchists believe in and practice.

As you wander through these pages, my hope is that you'll think for yourself, drawing out the theoretical insights that can only come from the lived activities of those who are acting as if social relations within our social experiments matter too. Because at this juncture of profound abandonment and horrifying scenes of barbarism, they do matter, if we are to both survive and thrive.

The stories stretch across varied landscapes and contexts, with different pieces emphasizing different dimensions of an anarcha-feminist praxis, which when brought together in conversation, paint a full(er) picture. Anthologies, to my mind, are about facilitating and holding a communal space for dialogue, in which we wrestle together with, to borrow the title from one of my previous books, "paths toward utopia." Key to this is the process itself, such as cultivating social relations with the contributors, or in the case of this project, supporting writer-rebels through the ways patriarchy socializes them to think their voices don't count. And trusting in people's lived experiences and storytelling as generative forms to unearth not just theory but hopefully change the world too—through our collective wisdoms. Indeed, I've come to see edited collections as a deeply feminist, anarchist, and queer practice (and a Jewish one, since ongoing, collaborative reinterpretation of the world through words is bound up in our duty to continually participate in trying to make the world whole through our actions).

The contributors in this book likewise share in their attention to "tending to the sparks" as a deeply feminist, anarchist, and queer practice. They offer their lived experiences as a small sample of those multitudes of "little" fire-keeping tasks that are too often discounted as "women's" (or marginalized genders') work, but without which nothing could burst forth into the "big" flames of revolution that allow us, if only for a divine duration, to "decide for ourselves" within free and autonomous time-spaces. Activist-writer Dilar Dirik—using storytelling as a method in another anthology—captured this magical relation between the embers of "women, life, freedom" combusting into the anarchically feministic region called Rojava:

> And one day,
> the (r)evolution came.
> We held instructions in our mighty hands,
> but the blueprints of the new era were pink and green and upside down,
> written in a language that none of us could read,
> except a mother with three kids on her back and five hiding under her skirt.
> "It says," she said,
> "don't expect from the gods, whether earthly or heavenly, what you can find in yourself."
> And thus, walked off

the illiterate woman,

to wash her face with the rays of the sun.[6]

These days, we must lean in close to feel the warmth of the "rays of the sun" against the coldness sweeping over this planet—a chill that finds its source in patriarchy, heteronormativity, and misogyny, even if it goes by other names like militarism and fascism, police and prisons. But those shimmering rays are there, in abundance, because of us, as you'll see in myriad ways on the pages ahead.

Against the backdrop of the collective trauma and systematic violence of the present era—when human and nonhuman life don't seem to matter at all, from Palestine to Turtle Island and beyond—those brilliant rays are there in the galaxies of communally caring practices, such as the ones so powerfully shared here, that intentionally strive to cultivate well-being, safety through solidarity, trust and friendship, vulnerability and consent, tenderness, reciprocity, accessibility, kindness, and so, so much more. They are there in innumerable on-the-ground projects that explicitly orbit around organizing as if social relations matter, illuminating how the future we dream of, even if unknown in the best possible sense, is already unfolding through fluid, expansive processes of tending lovingly to each other. They are there in our feministic, queered, anarchic, plain-old extraordinary, badass brave spaces, self-organized in kitchens and cafés, social centers and social uprisings, parks and theaters, solidarity apothecaries

---

6. Dilar Dirik, "'Only with You, This Broom Will Fly': Rojava, Magic, and Sweeping Away the State Inside of Us," in *Deciding for Ourselves: The Promise of Direct Democracy*, ed. Cindy Milstein (Chico, CA: AK Press, 2020), 201.

and collective clinics, schools and jail support, private living rooms and public squats—freely supplying an entire universe, materially and immaterially, of everything for everyone, until all are free.

December 13, 2023
Asheville, NC

❋  ❋  ❋

What you'll find between the covers of *Constellations of Care* is only a fraction of the many stories that were shared with me since I put out a "call" for pieces after Libertie Valance, with Firestorm bookstore, offhandedly suggested the idea of a contemporary anthology related to anarcha-feminism way back in summer 2021. (Shoutout and love to Libertie for her dear friendship, ability to generatively nudge my thinking, and contribution herein.) This book was, to my surprise, a fitful journey—more so than any other collection I've birthed. To my sorrow, patriarchy, including within anarchism, is so alive and well, it convinces way too many people that their experiences, ideas, and projects have no value, and that they can't or shouldn't write.

That translated into me scouring the globe numerous times, attempting to counter-convince feministic anarchists to tell their own stories—frequently without success. It translated into many, many dozens of anarchistic feminists getting in touch with sketches of what they wanted to explore or compelling full drafts, yet who alas couldn't get past the pain, understandably, of what anarcho-patriarchy had done to them in order to portray the beauty of own their practices (the aspiration of this book), or even find and believe in their own voices—despite my best efforts to lend as much support, encouragement, and collaborative aid as possible. To each and every one of you whose writing ultimately didn't appear here, I offer my gratitude, love, and solidarity; without you, without our many conversations, this book would not have materialized. You're on these pages in spirit.

I want to acknowledge as well the many friends, accomplices, and comrades who widely shared my call for contributions and translated it into Spanish, sent me contacts for potential writers and stories, generously supplied me with house+cat sits and thus time to write and edit, offered a listening ear, read through parts of the manuscript, wrote a blurb, and so much more—too many people to name by name, lest I forgot someone. Without you, without this social fabric of collective care "work," voluntarily given and gratefully received, this anthology would never have made it into the world. I trust you know who you are, and how much your love and solidarity means to me—love and solidarity that radiates across these pages because of you.

That said, I'd be remiss if I didn't name a few names— people who went many miles beyond what they likely thought they were "signing up for" when I turned to them for anarchist assistance. My heartfelt thanks to Steven, Erica Lagalisse, and Scott/Shuli Branson for their honest and supportive reflections as well as publishing expertise in helping me ultimately decide to go with Pluto Press. Much appreciation to Lilli Sher for reading and offering suggestions on my essay for this collection. Abiding gratitude to someone who is wholly—and always so beautifully—a collaborator on, now, the majority of my books: Jeff Clark of Crisis; his cover design captures the heart of this anthology, perhaps because his big heart so clearly bursts forth in what he dreamed up. And I hardly know how to begin to thank Wren Awry and Scott Campbell, much less complete any sort of appreciation for both of them. They traveled with me through the entire process of this volume. Their contributions herein are only the proverbial tip of the iceberg of what they gifted me, from being solid sounding boards, to empathetically supporting me through self-doubt on this project, to being dear friends who also write and publish, and so really got the depth of the waters when they shared their good counsel. Much love to you all.

To name other names, it's been an utter pleasure to work with Pluto Press, including from the first moment I met my Pluto editor, David Shulman, on a bench outside a conference he was attending in Montreal in summer 2023. He took a break to ostensibly chat with me briefly about this book, and we talked for over three hours about everything under the sun, from politics to life—except this project. David felt a kindred spirit from the get-go, and along with his belief in and enthusiasm for this anthology, he's made publishing a delight. Perhaps most important, he was there when I hit obstacles that made me feel I'd never finish this book, supplying just the right—and insightful—advice to aid me in moving forward. Abundant appreciation, too, to everyone I've worked with at Pluto—all of whom have been supportive, communicative, and eminently good at what they do: Chris Browne, Carrie Giunta, Geraldine Hendler, Patrick Hughes, James Kelly, Jonila Krasniqi, Sophie O'Reirdan, Emily Orford, Melanie Patrick, Martin Pettitt, and Robert Webb.

Lastly, my love extends to each and every contributor. I cannot express my gratitude enough for so beautifully and publicly sharing so much of yourselves and the splendor of your lived experiences in this book. That takes courage, and as your stories attest, walking the walk even when the going is lonely or tough. I'm in such admiration of your ability to remain true to your ethics, self-reflective, and openhearted— and not give up; instead, you just keep using your praxis as a bolt cutter to liberate more space for commons of care to emerge. It was an honor, moreover, to witness the many ways you all fully held to your feminist anarchist practices during our lengthy back-and-forths to go from idea through various stages of revisions to polished piece. So much struck me in that regard during our private exchanges, but I was especially moved by your commitment to and humility around uplifting collectivity; it feels a deeply anarcha-feminist action, as evidenced in every chapter, to unflinchingly believe that it takes many rebel voices—indeed all of our voices—to speak a new world into existence.

Cindy Barukh Milstein (they, or he, but never she) curates anthologies as labors of love and containers of possibilities.[7] As interventions so as to encourage a prefigurative politics, not merely one of negation. As inspiration to keep going toward infinite forms of collective freedom via messy-beautiful experimentation. As mirrors onto other possible worlds and lives that we're already enacting, even if only in glimpses. They do that as a queer diasporic Jewish anarchist, as a "street intellectual," at cross-purposes with all the ways that thinking has gotten separated from doing (and feeling) as yet another form of hierarchy and control. They do that as someone who has long tried hard to embody their ethics in practice, whether in their organizing, solidarity efforts, books, curation of magical time-spaces, love, or life. You can find Milstein on Instagram @cindymilstein, via cbmilstein.wordpress.com, or at cbmilstein@yahoo.com.

7. All author proceeds from this book will be redistributed to various anarcha-feminist initiatives, based on suggestions from the contributors to this collection and shifting with each round of royalties.

# THE COLLECTIVE AS A CRUCIAL FORM

/

TAHEL AXEL, ELIAS LOWE,
AMI WEINTRAUB,
LEO WILLIAMSON-REA,
AND FLIP ZANG

We are not writing this because we have something new to offer with our story.

Instead, like many young anarchists, we started out overflowing with hope and rage. We were fed up with a world that had been violent toward our bodies, a world represented by our rapists, the alt-right personalities doing campus speaking tours, the university chancellor with over a half-million-dollar salary who turned the other cheek when those Nazis came to town, the police who beat up our friends at protests and continued to kill Black people in the streets, and an increasingly fascist government with its different presidential faces.

Fed up, wounded, angry, scared, disillusioned. We had this in common, and it was not original, but it did feel powerful.

In fall 2015, when Nightshade had its first meeting—which was not really a meeting but rather a circle of outcasts telling stories in Ami's living room—we all had the same five Crimethinc posters on our walls, held up by peeling masking tape.[1] Back then, it was hard for some of us to even speak of the traumas we had experienced, and even harder to articulate our desires and fears.

But we were radicalized by the notion that we could become stronger together. At that first meeting, there were around twenty-five people packed into the little room. We went on to organize together for a while that autumn, not quite ever fulfilling our early dreams of crashing frat parties and beating up any cis men who were violating people's

---

1. *Editor's note:* It's a sweet coincidence that Nightshade is the name of two, albeit unrelated, collectives in this anthology (see "Tarps and Gossip").

consent, escorting girls and gay boys safely back to their homes, and being a sort of vigilante crew of queers who would keep each other safe when no one else would. Certainly, though, we found other ways of being brave in unison.

We did a lot of assembling and disrupting and empowering, grieving and experimenting and loving, as well as we knew how. Many of the people present at that initial meeting would go on to get retraumatized in one way or another. The year 2016 was full of ugly street protests and face-offs with bigots, followed by a scary wave of state repression. There were also a fair number of misogynists within the movement who claimed to be different, but in fact were insidious in their own ways, hurting us when we were most vulnerable.

It was clear to us then, as it is now, that anarchism needs feminism because misogynists make great informants, or because misogynists break up movements without even needing to be hired by the state since the state can rely on us hurting each other and being already too hurt for there to be a possibility for recourse.

The Nightshade collective continued to grow into itself, although it looked a lot different after its first year. Those of us still left over decided we would attempt to slowly change the culture of organizing through our creation of revolutionary, queer feminist content and by radically changing the way we treated one another. We hosted study groups on consent and radical conflict resolution, organized workshops and skill shares, made zines to spell out our pain and conjure moments for collective healing, participated in solidarity actions and night marches, held safe and sexy trans-positive dance parties, fostered intergenerational queer spaces where trans kids and elderly dykes and everyone in between could break bread, and engaged in immeasurable hours of interpersonal and relational work with one another. Inspired by the *tekmil* method utilized by revolutionaries in Rojava, we integrated strategies for giving and receiving feedback into our meetings and day-to-day relational cadences, believing thoroughly in the militancy of our love for each other to keep us accountable to our actions, develop our strengths as courageous and critical people, and ultimately sustain and expand the collective well-being.

Over our four years of existence, many of us "came out" as different versions of queer or trans, realizing ourselves anew with the support of the collective, which brought gender and sexuality into view as both deeply personal and potentially revolutionary, transformative, and playful when experimented with in a group. We joked that Nightshade was a she/they to they/he, or he/they to they/she pipeline.

It was easier to imagine a queer adult life for ourselves with all of our friends surrounding us and participating too. Leo's house was where Flip got their first "adult" queer hair cut in 2017, a collaboration between J and B, also in Nightshade back then, in front of the bathroom mirror. It was in that same living room that M told us their new name. We all cheered. Every week it seemed like there was another reason to celebrate the new parts of ourselves that we finally felt safe enough to explore and reveal.

We took our aspirations so seriously that we formally facilitated "dreaming sessions" where we would produce mind maps on large pieces of white paper detailing the worlds we were building. One of our goals was to "become serious contenders in the realm of anarchist theory and thought"—a desire to slash the gatekeeping and hierarchy of what *serious contenders* meant. Us queers without PhDs or refined "masculine" intellect could contribute too, and were contributing, just by virtue of gathering and refusing to stay silent.

It was important to us—and still is—to view our collective self-actualization as trans and queer subjects as a crucial intervention in the naturalization of cisheteropatriarchy and the violence it commands. We didn't want to "substitute some other great feminist truth for the great white masculinist truth," as Kim TallBear put it so eloquently. We were "trying to get it less wrong."[2] We were embracing our transness and queerness, and viewing them as a way to delegitimize an entire logic of oppressive domination and control (and not the sexy kind).

"Why is the transsexual or transgender subject to be explained, rather than the cissexual or cisgender one?" observed Xandra Metcalfe.[3] In many ways, Nightshade externalized this question through our very existence. To the local anarchist scene, to the University of Pittsburgh where many of us met as students, to the city and world at large, we strived to throw everything people thought they knew as objective and inherent about gender into doubt. Nightshade

---

2. Kim TallBear, "On Reviving Kinship and Sexual Abundance," *For the Wild* (podcast), episode 157, accessed December 5, 2023, https://forthewild.world/listen/kim-tallbear-on-reviving-kinship-and-sexual-abundance-157.

3. Xandra Metcalfe, "'Why Are We Like This?': The Primacy of Transsexuality," in *Transgender Marxism*, ed. Jules Joanne Gleeson and Elle O'Rourke (London: Pluto Press, 2021), 219.

wanted to shift the dominant assumption that heterosexuality and cisgenderism is natural, recognizing that fallacy as an epistemological imposition that we as trans subjects, or anyone for that matter, did not consent to—and have every right to reject.

So again and again, Nightshade came together in adamant refusal of all that failed to affirm us. We placed stickers over the gendered bathroom signs at Pitt so many times that the actual placards were removed from the walls. We took ourselves seriously despite outside skepticism, such as people (often cis dudes from "the scene") asking why we even existed in the first place. We defied the privacy of individual romantic partnerships and grounded ourselves in the intimate bond of queer friendship.

Though we were a queer and trans collective, we strove to go beyond the boundaries of identity politics and access the transformative capacity of raging against conformity in our everyday lives. By confronting moments of interpersonal conflict within our collective, we braced for the larger confrontations we would face as dissidents against the death mechanisms of white supremacy and capital.

No, we were not original, and we were also nowhere near perfect. We are not writing this because we think there is something necessarily new about our story, as we noted earlier; in fact, there is something wonderfully redundant going on here. When we were feeling insurmountably lonely, scared, and hurt, we formed a collective, and as that collective we created many temporary commons, and held each other and learned together and allowed ourselves to be militantly joyful, which sometimes looked like flipping the table of the campus Republicans (shoutout to T) or screaming in the faces of neofascist men, but more often looked like 2.5-hour meetings in the dead of winter circled around a pot of tea. All of that is worth talking about because we are all still here; in many ways it kept us alive, that collective form, and it kept us believing in a world that is vastly different than this one.

We learned to solidify the commons of care in fall 2018, when Brett Kavanaugh's confirmation process for a US Supreme Court seat turned into a public hearing on sexual assault. Kavanaugh was taken to task by the women he had harmed. The hearing made a spectacle of what we already knew: that patriarchal violence is a function of the state and therefore the state will never protect us from it. We knew this testimony would open wounds for many people who'd been raped, and decided that regardless of the outcome, we'd make care packages for anyone reliving trauma because of the hearing.

Over one hundred people requested packages in the first couple of days, and we began compiling emotional-resourcing zines, stickers, fidget toys, personalized cards, candles, and soaps, and delivering them to people both in Pittsburgh and across the United States. While we hoped to supply some relief to the survivors who responded to our offer, the ritual of giving care also helped keep us grounded and allowed us to move through our own grief. We discovered that in spite of the trendy online push toward an alienated framework for "self-care," people were desperately seeking a sense of togetherness, to be a part of a process of healing-in-common.

We found many feminist ways of surrounding each other. Sometimes it took the form of publicly calling out the names of our abusers while reveling in our collective sorrow and rage, or engaging in a circle of song in the middle of the street to hold a pain that is larger than life. At other times the care was gentle; it was medicine and healing spells and hugs. And then there was dancing; a queer dance party with a good DJ is enough to make time stop.

Nightshade's dance party fundraisers were always messy and fun. We decorated the walls of what was then the Glitterbox Theater with posters of our chosen trans ancestors. We spent hours experimenting with mixology, and coming up with cocktails and mocktails that sometimes tasted good and often tasted bad. We explored what it meant to feel "safe" at a party, and what it looked like to hold space in and with our bodies.

People of all ages would show up to the functions we hosted, and we took pleasure in the beauty and discomfort of intergenerationality. We danced with that discomfort, asked ourselves who was there, who was not there, and why. We received criticism. We also received a lot of positive feedback and gratitude from people who told us they had never felt so held before, whether at a dance party, event, meeting, or meal.

We hear "care work" thrown around a lot these days, and because it's not "productive" labor, it's impossible to really measure the results. But something Nightshade learned early on was that it didn't matter if our success was measurable so long as it was feeling right, so long as there was someone who was on the receiving end of a gift. The rituals we created together could not be boxed into the logistic flow of capitalism. What did "right" feel like? Incompletion, abundance, joy, sustenance, time travel.[4] A flower opening up and embracing the light. There is nothing to do with beauty but be present in it—and wait in wonderment for the fleeting thing to fade.

Incompletion and flexibility carried us through countless transitions and formations.

We learned this most clearly in fall 2018, when several organizers of color in Pittsburgh expressed concern that our whiteness was impacting our practices in ways that hurt Black and Brown people. In light of this, we decided to slow down our public organizing and focus on internal antiracism education facilitated by an outside organization as well as one another. In hindsight, we have different perspectives about this time period and could not fully agree on how to talk about it in this piece. This lack of uniformity speaks to the complexity of identity politics, callout culture, and organizing in a white supremacist world. We were beginning to discuss how to move forward as a collective when the pandemic hit.

We met for the last time without knowing it would be the last time. We had different ideas of what would feel necessary and what we had capacity to do together in the face of a new type of crisis and emergency. We were not sure how to envision a future together as Nightshade and perhaps knew in our hearts that it was time—time for a collective that was once beautiful to disperse and learn from our many messy conflicts

---

4. À la Stefano Harney and Fred Moten, incompletion means to resist the impulse to constantly improve, and then constantly manage and own what you improve on. Instead, we aim to simply be all that we share and what we lose happily through sharing, which is our completeness, the possibility of our ever being finished, staying smugly uncontainable. Stefano Harney and Fred Moten, *All Incomplete* (London: Minor Compositions, 2021).

as our politics had instructed us to do. We began gathering our energy for pressing and diverse mutual aid projects, and continued growing our relationships elsewhere, but without abandoning each other as friends.

Even with the imperfections of Nightshade, over those four years we formulated a model for community care amid a landscape of trauma and gendered violence. That care sustained our relationships through attacks that could've easily broken us apart beyond repair. We cultivated an anarchist feminist vision together that we continue to scatter like seeds.

These seeds take the form of questions—questions we carry forward into our new projects and relationships: How can we better apply feminist care to form loving bonds across all the lines that racial capitalism uses to devastate and divide us? How can we build collectives that withstand the punitive culture imposed by elite capture? How do we continue to queer resistance, queer time, and wreck capitalism through our very existence as well as our love for one another?

Two years after the last official Nightshade meeting, five of us gathered in a cabin on a snowy mountain in West Virginia. We still find each other on occasions such as this to sing songs, play games, and dream up the endless possibilities for revolt. We still love each other as chosen family.

Perhaps this story has no precise point, or perhaps it is simply evidence that the collectives we make with our friends are important manifestations of anarchist feminism, and we must honor them in all of their complicated fits and starts. The collective form is a crucial part of how we gather. It will be messy and generative, and most important, it will not be forever, and that will come with uncertainty and grief. But death work, like birth work, has always been the work of women, trans people, and queers.

As anarchists and abolitionists in the midst of worldwide ecological and social catastrophe, *we need a trans feminist practice*. This is to say we need a practice of self and collective transformation that ties us deeply into interdependent webs with one another. We need a process that teaches us how to let go of all that we cannot take into new worlds and allows us to mourn all that the old world has taken from us. We need the queer wisdom of knowing how to transition, change, and grieve. We can only rest on our intangible knowing, the silent spaces our words don't always fill. This growing intuition hums with immutable vibration.

Yes, this is an argument for the anarchist feminist collective as a form. And this is a solidarity statement with all the women and queers internationally, from Iran to Serbia and back to Turtle Island, whose bodies and spirits are forced to endure the ongoing violence of patriarchy. And this is a call for the defense of the commons and the construction of new ones worldwide, wherever and whenever possible. This is a love story of five to twenty-five queer friends who at various moments believed the worlds we were creating together had the power to dismantle empires. This is a letter of gratitude, to all who participated in Nightshade as collective members as well as the people who came to our events, those who critiqued us, and those who came before us and inspired us to act.

May we continue to embrace the irrationality of dreams, joy of surprise, soundness of ritual, and method of creating new cultures of care and revolutionary practice through playful rehearsal. May we continue to have faith in the supernatural, the earth, and each other, and always fight for and with the magic of life despite attempts around us to kill it. We hope there is something for you in this story too.

❊　❊　❊

This essay is the product of many months of reconnecting, remembering, and discussion. The words were written by Flip with essential contributions from Tahel, Elias, Ami, and Leo.

Tahel Axel (they/them) feels most at home hiking in big mountains, and while making Shabbat with friends and loved ones. They love spending time in the overgrowth of postindustrial Pittsburgh, where they currently reside. Tahel is working toward becoming a midwife and dreams of dismantling the multilayered oppressions of our current "health care" system.

Elias Lowe is a writer, student of natural medicine, and committed friend currently living in Berlin. They spend their time seeking connection with people and lands, and searching for abolition in the everyday. They try to stay kind while raging against the death of the planet. Elias thanks their comrades and loves in Pittsburgh who grew them into a person who is able to survive.

Ami Weintraub (he/they) is a Jewish anarchist writer and rabbinic student. Ami's work and community organizing focus on building a world without domination where people can freely connect to their cultures, lands, and bodies. They call the hills of Pittsburgh and creeks of Silver Spring, Maryland, home.

Leo Williamson-Rea (they/he) feels most at home near water and loves the chaos magic of rerooting relationality. In between mischief and healing, Leo enjoys spending time with plants, singing songs in the moonlight, and learning different means of defending what they love.

Flip Zang (he/him) is a writer and geohistorian born and raised in Shawanwaki/Shawnee and Osage land (also known as Pittsburgh). He likes to make music and ask big questions, and can never decide which thing to love most.

# OUR AFFINITY IS OUR MANIFESTO

/

MEXICO CITY–BASED
FEMINIST-ANARCHIST
AFFINITY GROUP IN
CONVERSATION WITH
AND TRANSLATED
BY SCOTT CAMPBELL

*Greetings, compas! Thanks for agreeing to talk with me. How would you like to introduce yourselves?*

We should start by saying that we aren't a collective or formal group. We see ourselves more as a small group of women and nonconforming folks who are united by love, friendship, and the struggle for freedom, autonomy, mutual aid, and life against the dynamics of the current patriarchal state. We come from different anarchist positions and understand things differently in many cases, but we come together to do things jointly based on trust and the need to support our existence. We live in different parts of Mexico City, where we carry out most of our struggles.

Or to put it more poetically, we are women of all the fires, born in lands full of misery. Our lives are written in the wind, and our struggles, loves, longings, and desires to change this reality live in the sea, in the waves that beat furiously on the rocks that contain them. Each one of us has her own history, forged with smiles and tears. Each one walks alone, yet we are strengthened by our paths that unite with the libertarian idea. Our hair is interwoven, and we move forward together, trying to be a support, company, and embrace, despite everything, despite the uncertainty and this overwhelming moment, despite the repression.

Survivors of the terrible, only the wind will know the passion with which we once tried, at some moment, in some time, for humanity to be strengthened by the beauty of mutual cooperation and disobedience, without states, exchanges, competition, and capitalism.

*Can you share with us how you came to your anarcha-feminist positions, how you found one another, and how you decided to form an affinity group?*

Not all of us conceive of ourselves as anarcha-feminists. We're all anarchists, antiauthoritarians, and antipatriarchal, yet we've never arrived at having a joint identity. We came together based on the recognition that our own experiences have provided. We're a group that ranges from twenty to forty years old. As such, we don't all have the same paths, trajectories, or positions.

All of our stories are individual ones, and each one took its time. For some, what was important was the break with those men who we believed to be compañeros, but who betrayed, hurt, or snitched on us. With that we saw the crumbling of a discourse that was just that: a discourse—and one that didn't delve deeply into how patriarchy runs through us. For others of us, the reality of being women and feminized bodies was always present: how we weren't listened to or were made invisible in political anarchist spaces; that only masculine voices were respected; and that even when we sustained various activities and a large part of the anarchist movement in the city, we continued to be relegated to the margins and unheard. So we assumed a position of defense and necessary confrontation within the movement, which was exhausting, but that helped us to be in this place today, together.

In a way, we lost our fear of separatism [femme-only spaces], although we never stopped seeing that there are men in this world we would have to interact with. We found one another in mixed, anarchist movement spaces through that recognition of oppressions intertwined with gender, class, schooling, age, and others. Sometimes this process of encounter was simultaneous to our male "compañeros" dropping like flies due to reports of sexual or physical aggression against other compañeras, which we could not deny or support. We were left in a space limited to mostly femme bodies where sisterhood and recognition occurred among peers and through our own experiences. We were left alone, or rather, we were defining our affinities with greater judgment—how great! We recovered our affinity as feminized bodies within the anarchist struggle. We recognized ourselves as survivors.

From there, the confluence of our actions keeps us together. We fully trust each other regarding our position with respect to the state and the police, for example. We also know that each one of us walks the path of self-management, and not hand in hand with NGOs [nongovernmental organizations] or human rights groups. This has given us much of the confidence and trust that we have—even though, we repeat, we don't all come from the same anarchist background. We are united in our belief that our unwavering principles are an essential part of our ethics.

*What are your perspectives on the resurgent feminist movement in so-called Mexico that began in 2018?*

Although the "boom" in the feminist movement around the world became more visible in the media in 2018, with massive marches on March 8, strikes in universities in Chile, Mexico, Spain, France, Italy, the United States, and so on, we hold that previous struggles can't be left out of this upsurge. Whether we like them or not, that includes approaches that we don't adopt—as seen, for example, in the proabortion discourses that push for legislative and constitutional changes. We believe that the struggle for the reappropriation of our bodies marks an indisputable precedent; in some countries, the voices of women and other bodies are beginning to be heard, and the struggle for the right to decide for ourselves is strengthening. And not just with respect to abortion but also with respect to individual decisions around sexual pleasure.

In the case of Mexico and specifically Mexico City, the struggle was obscured, as it was appropriated by the state and leftist government. The existence of a small oasis in this country that provides noncriminalized abortion and guarantees for gay persons loses force due to the state's interference in women's bodies. For us, it is not enough for the state to decriminalize abortion, we simply and plainly do not want it to be in charge of regulating our sexuality and controlling our bodies.

Yet it is true that in Mexico, we live in a very particular situation that makes this boom urgent and inevitable. We're talking about the fact that in our territory, more than eleven women are killed every day. A boom that, we must also recognize, arrived late. What are we referring to? To the murders on the northern border, in Ciudad Juárez, where the neologism *femicide* was born during the 1990s. Why didn't the feminist boom explode then? Why was the massive murder of working women on the border made invisible? Why were we not outraged by so many bodies found scattered around the desert?

It's true that those were different times, and many of us were children or had not yet been born. Nevertheless, we believe that it goes beyond that; that it has to do with women whose deaths did not "deserve" to cause indignation because they were socially and morally devalued by the hegemonic discourse. They were morally unacceptable for going out late at night, for going out alone. They were invalidated under the construction of bodies that simply do not matter: poor, from the periphery, and workers. The state was lucky that there wasn't enough social courage for the entire country to erupt at that point in the fight against death. Of course, at that time there were feminist collectives, academics, and some politicians who pointed out the need to look at this problem. But we have to recognize that the state won that fight when, to this day, we're not even able to remember the names of some of these women, when we find it hard to say that we didn't see or know what to do and that the state imposed its version of history. Unfortunately, the so-called feminist boom can be read as an urgency to respond to the femicides of less stigmatized bodies too—university students, professionals, middle-class mothers, and so on—and it is equally regrettable that even in this situation, the same categories are still used to determine who gets named and who doesn't, such as the poor, whores, workers, and single mothers.

We like to think that the feminist boom is not 2018 and nothing more, that women and feminized bodies don't only appear when the media and government decide to "recognize us." We like to think that we can honor our ancestors by giving continuity to a struggle that we have joined, that we did not originate, and that doesn't answer to external agendas or media attention but rather to an inevitable necessity where we fight to stay alive and not forget any of our dead.

*Street actions get a lot of attention, but beyond those, how have you all been involved in the broader feminist movement?*

As we've mentioned, we're not a formal group, much less a homogeneous one, and therefore the ways in which we're involved in the feminist movement are equally diverse. Some of us accompany the anticarceral struggle, in which some compañeras have faced charges after participating in feminist actions or protests; others of us are involved in graphic design, which continues to be necessary to visualize the struggle in the streets and online; others are committed to physical self-defense; others of us contribute through print publishing; others are committed to radio work; yet others are involved in the self-management of mental and physical health; others have started and sustain spaces of resistance such as bookstores, libraries, and cooperatives; and others are involved in solidarity economies. In general, we're all in search of life and survival, which basically robs us of a lot of time and energy.

Something that has become necessary to do together, though, has to do with the precarious conditions that most feminized bodies experience. In this regard, in 2020 [when the pandemic began], we saw how women were at greater risk due to the forced confinement because they were with their aggressors all the time. It was necessary to go out and call on women to fight for life and occupy the streets. We called for the creation of small markets, flea markets, and bazaars by and for women—there were also trans and queer friends—with the idea of surviving by exchanging the products we made and to spread awareness about our self-managed projects.

The organizing that has occurred since the pandemic has allowed for the opening of furrows where we've seen self-management and rebellion flourish, and where we've brushed its fierce and faint breath with anarchy. That's how we found ourselves in the streets within a broader feminist movement. This is not easy because there are many positions and understandings within the movement that we don't necessarily coincide with, but we firmly believe that it is the differences that make us powerful.

We believe that maintaining a fierce and voracious critique against the state and capitalism permits us to not waste time betting on lost struggles—for instance, for the approval of laws that guarantee us security that in the majority of cases, are applied against us or help to criminalize what is already criminalized: the poor and racialized. But we also see that especially in our context, in certain struggles, our critique isn't applicable—for example, the struggles undertaken by the mothers of the disappeared or murdered. We don't see ourselves as having the ability or arrogance to tell them not to seek "justice" from within institutions or not to engage in dialogue with the representatives of power, because there are many cases where that is impossible to avoid. On the contrary, we see ourselves as deeply inspired by them, by their actions and paths. We believe that it is those collectives that nourish us and give us a lot of strength to continue.

*How would you describe your own general orientation when taking action?*

As we come from anarchism, and we have little by little been breaking with its classical vision of struggle, we understand that the struggle is found in all spaces, micro and macro. Therefore we don't see the need to wait for some moment to intervene in this or that; rather, we believe in the necessity of placing strain on the relations of domination—among them gender and sex—in the spaces that we inhabit: families, collectives, compañerxs, and ourselves. But we can't do that if we don't struggle to make it clear that we exist, to make a space for ourselves among the already established structures of struggle, dissent, and society in general. That same space gives us the opportunity to make our positions clear, to go forward as we would like to live and according to our principles—that is, outside the institutions, away from the state, through direct action, self-management, and autonomy.

Contrary to the fashion of "visibility," we position ourselves through obscure and opaque daily action. Our action is our own manifesto.

*Speaking of taking action, what has your experience of participating in feminist actions felt like, and what has it made possible that previously might have seemed foreclosed to you?*

A point of street action that seemed impossible was the acceptance of the slogan "It was all of us" in a moment when the white feminist discourse seemed to prevail and the supposedly citizenly idea of the "good feminist" kept appearing, almost to the point of them becoming the "police" of the demonstrations, which they actually did with a citizen call to protect women police officers during the protests under the argument that they were also "sisters" and "women."[1] Currently, this slogan has been taken up by more and more compañeras in the street, and that is motivating, but we'd still like to transcend the slogan, and see criminalization and political correctness be challenged. Even so, hearing in unison "It was all of us," and taking on the rage of others as our own, brings the body joy and reaffirms our presence in the streets.

We were not enlightened by 2018, so to speak. Many of us had already traveled a long road in the anticapitalist and autonomous struggle. It was anarchy that gave us the possibility to position ourselves from a place of autonomy and have a deep critique of what it is to struggle against the prevailing system of domination. This path has given us immense possibilities, necessary stumbles, and inevitable ruptures. We have learned that from all of this, self-criticism, pressures, and openings emerge. One opening was perhaps feminism, which has swayed us with respect to many questions, leading us to explore micro- and infrapolitical spaces. We approach feminism to a greater or lesser extent and make critical distinctions because we're not convinced that there is only one feminism, nor do we try to pursue it.

To place the body [in action] is, in this sense, to assume our struggle from within ourselves and toward the outside. To embody [feminist] struggle is to realize that part of it

---

1. "Fuimos todas" (It was all of us) was a slogan used in response to the direct actions carried out during feminist mobilizations. Instead of pointing out those responsible for the actions to the police, everyone chanted their complicity.

corresponds with us, such that we suffer and are not indifferent to it. The somatic experience of this is indistinct from all we're doing. Sometimes we are literally a ticking time bomb, and sometimes we're bodies that are vulnerable. Sometimes we are filled with collective strength, and other times we feel like weirdos and that we're singled out to such a degree that we become tiny. Sometimes we laugh out loud, and at other times we simply weep in torrents.

*What has it meant for you all to be an affinity group of feminist anarchists participating in the movement and being there for each other as opposed to going it alone?*

We go alone and together. We believe in each other's individuality and the power of being together. But we know that not all of us want or can take on the same things, or have the same abilities, to mention a few differences. Even so, knowing that we exist as a rare and amorphous entity has given us security in moving about our city. We know that if one of us falls into the clutches of the police, there will be many of us outside the police station or prison entrance. We know that if one of us is sick, we'll have another one accompanying and caring for us. And we know that whatever idea we want to carry out, we can share it and find an echo among others.

In this way, we see that affinity cannot be measured entirely in political, strategic, and pragmatic terms but instead goes hand in hand with how it transcends and traverses love, friendship, and the struggle for survival. Are we in affinity? Yes, but we are also accomplices, sisters, friends, and compañeras. We don't just see ourselves as an affinity group or meet because of that. We do it because we care about each other's lives too, because we like to laugh together, eat together, cook together, and believe that this is how we'll be able to survive. This encourages us a lot.

*This is a broad question, but how do you articulate your own feminist anarchism?*

As we mentioned, we have different roots, and sexuality has not affected each of us in the same way and that means many things. The older members of our group grew up in a fairly heterosexual anarchist scene, and therefore nonconformity was more opaque or simply did not appear. Of course, we have precious beings who are openly gay, but we understand, as the anarchist scene here is heterosexual, that those bodies escape from those spaces and construct their own. We recognize that we came late to many criticisms in this sense, and little by little we have learned to come out of the closet ourselves or deconstruct our own sex-gender identity, although we don't see it as the core that defines us.

Indeed, we have a critique of identity. Sometimes it means taking on an essence in order to act from a certain positionality, but most of the time it blurs a series of differences that to us, seem necessary in order to walk together. Perhaps before indicating our sexual identity, we start from the point of being "dark-skinned" or Indigenous descendants—an inevitable matter that situates us on the stage of antagonistic struggles and more so in an essentially racist country. We are also poor; we come from places and families that have always struggled for survival.

We've learned that we can't generalize, even though there are structures that affect all of us. And in that sense, we see ourselves as distant from some groups of trans and nonbinary people because we don't share conditions of class or race. As we have grown up marked by that racism, there are many nonconforming spaces where we don't feel comfortable, or where that feeling of being seen as strange or exotic accompanies us. Many queer and nonconforming spaces—not all—are part of the art world, and we experience them as white and hostile places. Likewise, some of these people take part in the struggle from institutional, academic, or NGO spaces—spaces denied to us and that we reject. Our reality sometimes doesn't allow us to understand their direction, and many times we feel we don't share the same concerns. Maybe it has to do with us still struggling in a broader sense by not abandoning the enormous desire to destroy the state and see capitalism fall. Sometimes, the nonconforming compas focus a lot on the construction of sex and gender and our positions begin to bore them. Ha ha.

We don't take identity as the starting point—even though a few of us are nonconforming—but rather the practice and ethics of our political actions, and anarchism on some occasions has given us the answer to feeling comfortable with our sexual and political differences. We think it would be much better if anarchism were nourished by questions of gender and sexuality, and displaced the machismo and heteronormativity that lives in its core, just as anarchism can bring important questions to the queer and nonbinary struggles. In our ideal dream, this mutual reciprocity goes hand in hand.

We also know that language is patriarchal, so we take on the responsibility of thinking of new ways of naming ourselves, and we are learning to do so.

We don't trust cis men. Our space does not seek to directly link with these compañeros. We don't reject mixed spaces of work or coexistence, but our primary affinity is with women and feminized bodies, as we mentioned earlier. The relationship in mixed groups has almost always felt to us like a utilitarian one stemming from supposed collective and political positions. We're not interested in feeling threatened by or vulnerable to patriarchal thoughts.

Since the break with cis men in our spaces, we have seen a conscious organizational advance from the perspective of anarcha-feminism. Our presence in the streets and taking on demands from an antipatriarchal perspective have been fundamental to seeing and being in solidarity with others in different latitudes. Understanding that women around so-called Latin America are being murdered as a result of being objectified as merchandise has given us the opportunity to create spaces for dialogue to understand our realities. The radicalization of demonstrations has called on us to denounce and act against disappearances, femicides, and antiabortion.

Our affinity is not only because we are women or nonconforming; it is because in our actions, we seek a radical rupture with traditional patriarchal impositions and we see with pleasure that this rage is spreading, beginning transcendent struggles. In some countries, this has been initiated by women, and has been able to stay active due to organizational persistence that emanates from our groups or individualities.

As for our aspirations, the least we try to do is walk toward life in a dignified way, and toward death in a meaningful way, even if it's for ourselves. The maximum: social revolution, the destruction of the capitalist-patriarchal system, the creation of other forms of living life, although we're not married to the idea that someday this will appear; rather, we're building it as much as we can in the here and now.

❊ ❊ ❊

As for our informal affinity group, we have no names that define us. Only the knowledge that nature is everything and humanity is destruction. To change that is our path.

Scott Campbell is a radical writer and translator residing in both what they call the United States and Mexico. His personal website is fallingintoincandescence.com. For a longer version of this interview, visit itsgoingdown.org/feminist-anarchist-affinity-group-interview.

# TEA, BOOKS, AND THRESHOLDS

## /

CORINNE, AURORE,
ÉRIS, AND TOM

*Even though it is our fingers that hit the keyboard, the countless hours spent working, chatting, and organizing with our fellow anarcha-feminist librarians and broader network led to these words. True to our ways, we speak on nobody else's behalf, yet we recognize our deep interdependence and write with what we feel is the "spirit" of the whole group in mind.*

The Anarcha-Feminist Library of Toulouse, or Bibliothèque Anarcha-Féministe—fondly called la BAF, a wordplay on the French *baffe*, meaning "slap," or just la bibli—is a couple-thousand-book-rich self-organized library in a major city in the southwest of France. We rent a place, Au Chat Noir (At the Black Cat), together with four other organizations, including a chapter of an anarcho-syndicalist / revolutionary syndicalist union, a local anarchist group, an antifascist group, and an anarchist-communist group. Additional organizations, such as a trans support group, fat-positive feminist zine-making group, and discussion group against borders, are regular users of the space. The library is, in a way, the shop front of the building: whether you enter Au Chat Noir for an organizing meeting, movie night, or support group, you can't fail to notice the thousands of colorful books happily displayed on wooden shelves as well as the comfortable chairs, blankets, and rugs made for snuggling up with a novel and herbal tea. In practice, we're open on Wednesday and Sunday after-noons—recently, we've been opening on Friday afternoons too, for a special "quiet library session" during which we keep the space as silent as possible to make it accessible to people who are otherwise disturbed or impaired by chatty or noisy environments—with frequent book or feminism-related events in between. It's a fun and quite telling fact that when most activities are more or less paused during the summer in Toulouse, in summer 2022 we were actually open one extra afternoon per week, just because it's a nice place to hang out, chill, or work on personal projects, and those of us who were staying in Toulouse during those months were happy to spend yet another day at la BAF.

Borrowing books is free; we do not track or register borrowers, and don't set a time limit on how long people use a book (we just ask that people keep in mind that others might want to read the same book, and so remember to bring it back when finished or given up on). Taking books home is easy, as borrowers need only write the titles down in a notebook along with a name/alias and cross out the entries once they bring them back.

But let's not spoil everything for you in this intro! Dear reader, will you dare push the paper door of la BAF open and follow a few funky tea-and-vegan-cake-addicted, extroverted-introverted librarians down the path?

## HOW TO SET UP AN ANARCHA-FEMINIST LIBRARY

The library was born from the collision of a pile of books and a space.[1] It has changed and is still evolving with the people we've met along the way.

Books came first: via a kleptomaniac friend who plundered Toulouse's independent bookshops but had to move and leave some of their treasure behind, some gifts from families and friends, extra copies from other anarchist libraries, and a

---

1. This section was written by Corinne.

crowdfunding campaign to buy books on anarchist women when I was a student. As for the building, the local syndicalist union had lost its meeting space, and along with other anarchist and antifascist groups, floated the idea of renting a spot to be shared for our own projects, that of other like-minded collectives, and/or people from the neighborhood who might want to start a social center or host community activities.

I was part of one of these groups at the time, and initially we meant to manage the library as one of the collective features of the space. Many anarchist/revolutionary spaces in France have such a library, yet it often collects dust and isn't used much.

When the gilets jaunes (yellow vests) movement in France started in November 2018, it created a strong division in the group that I was part of (as it did in the wider anarchist movement) around whether and/or how to engage with this uprising. The gilets jaunes' struggle centered on the cost of living, and was driven at first largely by Far Right and conspiracist movements, although it then morphed into a class-based movement for dignity and against police violence. Interpersonal conflicts were added to the gilet jaunes' disagreements in my group, and we lost most of our members and then merged with another group.

I wasn't involved in the main debates around the gilets jaunes. I was rather critical of any kind of social movement premised on momentary bursts of intensity and simply pointing to the failures of structures like capitalism. For me at least, this wasn't a sustainable way to work toward liberation, especially because this recurring pattern feels both mentally and physically exhausting. I was more involved in dealing with the interpersonal conflicts, but it soon became apparent that beneath a superficial agreement on accountability and conflict resolution, our tools and principles were co-opted by certain people in our group to justify the unjustifiable and avoid challenging any of their own behaviors.

A few months later, I was no longer part of any group and yet didn't want to give up the efforts made in working with the different local groups to open a space.

When a shared space was rented, it started in the image of the "official" anarchist organizations in France—in particular, extremely male dominated—so despite my hesitations, I decided to help set it up. Having to work across organizational barriers forced me and everyone else to be more civil and accountable toward each other—to care more about others. The space appealed to me because I wanted a project on a longer timescale, with continuous yet limited effort (as opposed to movement building) for my own well-being. Then too, I wanted to focus on establishing strong, dependable, and honest interpersonal relationships by working directly and practically with other people, as opposed to taking positions in an abstract way as part of a group and caring more about how the group would be perceived by the rest of the revolutionary movement than about how we treated each other.

Once the library was created (as a project; we had not yet joined Au Chat Noir at this point), we thought about whether we wished to be a women-and-queer-only group and decided against it, although we were quite happy that our first public appeal had only been answered by women and queers. We then requested to join Au Chat Noir as a separate group—or at least to try, because I assumed that it wouldn't be easy to get the other groups in the space to tolerate this notion. What I didn't realize was how much these other groups needed people to do the actual job of making the space come alive—that is, by the women and queer people who showed up—and what they had to gain by having a "feminist" token group to share the overall project with.

Au Chat Noir invited us to a meeting to discuss the idea of us joining. There are at least two diverging accounts of how this meeting went. In my version, although I was upset at having to face the person who had driven me to quit my former group not long before, I expected little from the groups comprising the building. So when we were given the keys and a time slot to open the library, I was over the moon. We had approached other spaces, but none were as well fitted to what we had in mind. These other spaces were often sympathetic but private businesses where people would feel pressured into, say, paying for drinks and so on, when it was essential to us that our library shouldn't have this kind of setting. The version from the other three people goes like this: they were not enthused by the people who called us "comrades" (which is not a term that we ever used and was rather off-putting) and were still condescending despite their best efforts, but they decided not to challenge them as they knew I was tired of conflict.

We all remember that the meeting was way too long, running past the breaking of the fast for Ramadan, so we cut it short as politely as we could and drove to Kentucky Fried Chicken.

## THE DRAFTS OF BITTERNESS

Outside the time when the library was open, those of us with la BAF only communicated using the "Drafts" folder of an email address that all four of us had access to. What this meant was that when we received emails regarding Au Chat Noir's maintenance that were not always kind or caring, one of us would immediately draft a response that got saved in the "Drafts" folder, such that we could all edit along—in a crude, pre–Google Drive version of collaborative writing. Others would then add things such as "I can't believe they did this. ... But is telling them to fuck off a good approach strategically?" Then the email draft would either become a civil yet firm response, one edit at a time, or devolve into an outlet for us to vent about whatever was going on, creating a weird collage of anger, jokes, and political analysis that helped us cope with the (rare) negative experiences we encountered with other groups.

Sometimes we shied away from raising an issue because we were tired and felt discouraged at the prospect of writing our grievance down for others in the space. But it helped to share our feelings with each other in the early stages, focusing on what we wanted to achieve, and whether it was fair and reasonable or counterproductive, all things considered. More often than not, ranting in a draft email was sufficient, and allowed us to calm down and realize we had less to gain from stirring up an issue than we had in ignoring it and instead strengthening ourselves so as to proactively intervene in—and stop—similar occurrences in the future. Sometimes another form of action was taken: we wrote and shared a calmer email, or engaged in a face-to-face discussion; in a few instances, the drafts were polished into angry emails to individuals or groups in the space. In all cases, drafting emails to each other and talking about them collectively gave us time to reflect together, and take everyone's emotions, distress, and concerns into account, especially because many people found it easier to express themselves in writing. The "drafts of bitterness" were our way to hold space for our feelings while at the same time working together as a group away and up from feelings to political stances. It was a practice of community care, and helped us become wiser in when and how to raise concerns and take actions—even if it meant having a Pandora's box of spite and rage tucked away somewhere.

But let me return to the how-tos of our anarcha-feminist library.

## REARRANGING OUR SHELVES AND SELVES

The books we had at the beginning were mostly on the history of social movements and historical anarchist women. We wanted the library to be in tune with movements as they exist today and the issues they are dealing with. At that time in France, there was an emerging feminist theory that was against capitalism and the state, and advocated for the abolition of prisons. There was a will (strongly repressed by the government and media) to challenge French republican "universalism" and talk about racism. The queer and crip movements were also starting to publish their first books (zines and pamphlets already existed).

So we started collecting more feminist and queer books, particularly titles that seemed essential. We began attempting to decolonize the works in our library by being vigilant about what social movements we were still ignoring. At the same time, we wanted to offer novels, poetry, plays (which are just as political as nonfiction books), graphic novels (which are extremely popular and offer many testimonies of life on the margins), and books for younger people so as not to exclude anyone.

While all of that sounds easy enough, we've run into all sorts of dilemmas when aspiring to fill out our shelves. Or to put it another way, our library has taught us much about the world and ourselves—in generative ways that only aid la BAF in living up to its anarcha-feminism.

In terms of feminist books, here in France at least, feminism sells, and many mainstream publishers go along with this fad. Some great books are published, but also many ersatz ones, with any radical content expunged, meaning it's harder to find those with liberatory and/or anarchist content. For example, we haven't always known what to do about feminist second-wave classics, many of which have outdated, "problematic" content about race, transness, or sex work, to name a few. So we have regular discussions on books that offer "representation" only, but are not necessarily well written or have little radical content apart from presenting, say, queer characters (which is radical in itself given the publishing landscape in France). Our "process" for choosing books becomes most obvious when we receive some as gifts from visitors: many times we just sit around a pile of books none of us have read, skimming through the pages and glancing skeptically at the cover, pondering whether they are worth adding. Decisions are hard to make, and sometimes we excavate a pile of undecided-on books in the meeting room, a sign from past librarians failing to choose to keep or dump them. It mostly comes down to deciding by the "vibe" among us—and if a book is removed later because the vibe changes, so be it.

Then, too, reading Afro-feminist Fania Noël made us aware of a bias on our shelves: we had much more about Black liberation in the United States—such as works by Angela Davis and bell hooks—than in France and its (former) colonies. We had already had a similar discussion on how Emma Goldman is viewed as the one anarchist woman and we needed to correct that misperception by the titles we offered in our library. Each book, with its quotes and bibliography, made us discover more authors. And the journey goes on ...

When we started this task of decolonizing our space, I thought it was just about adding more diverse references. Only recently have I realized what should have been obvious all along: reading these books, relating to them critically, has changed my worldview, and how I consider social issues and sometimes even relate to people.

Questioning why hooks was one of the most requested and borrowed authors at our library, for instance, led me to understand that while her writings are precious in prefiguring a way to act together with men and across color lines, they also can be read as notions easy to accept on a superficial level, without changing much in the way we do things. Philosopher Norman Ajari, on the other hand, has done a tremendous amount of work in making Afro-pessimism known to French readers. From an anarchist point of view, Afro-pessimism reminds us that structures of power do not stop running through us only because we know how to name them; we need autonomous groups with enough power that they can't be disregarded in order to start envisioning as well as building a revolutionary movement together.

In Toulouse, the feminist and queer movements are close, and these interpersonal networks have meant that for a long time, the library has been run exclusively by LGBTQ people. A trans collective meets weekly in our space, for example, and makes the library available as part of the other services it offers. Queer literature is always in high demand.

Toulouse also has a number of antiableism and deaf groups. Our space is not yet accessible for wheelchair users (some wheelchair users have visited the space, but the conditions in which we welcome them are not satisfactory). We are working (extremely slowly) with the other groups in the building on accessibility issues, and have recently gathered enough books on these topics to fill a shelf on disability and deaf cultures. This is quite obviously the area, though, where most improvement is urgently needed.

### KEEPING THE DOORS OPEN

It has happened more than a few times that when I was talking about la BAF to someone, I preferred using the more politically neutral phrase "associative library," which in France refers to a community or nonprofit organization, instead of using "anarcha-feminist"—knowing that the overtly political name could lead to heated reactions.[2] Indeed, on a few occasions when I called la BAF by its name, I've been met with harsher reactions such as, "Oh, so you're one of those

---

2. This section was written by Aurore.

women yelling all tits out!" True story. Several of us have had similar experiences, reflecting the lack of knowledge or even awareness about feminist movements, or antagonism toward them.

There are, of course, many different ways to conduct the struggle, including by creating warm, welcoming spaces like la BAF. You don't have to protest loudly and bare chested, though that is certainly one of many ways to engage. To each their own ways to fight; to each their own ways to express and relate to resistance.

But how do we explain any of this to people not already in our circles? The activist milieu in Toulouse, however diverse and dynamic, remains relatively closed (which is also a way to protect ourselves, as we'll develop later). We run the risk of staying in a comfortable, familiar, secluded environment in which ideas circulate in a locked-in system among like-minded peers. It is thus necessary to find a balance between community protection and permeability.

That's why, in order to spread our ideas but also make the library and its activities known, a key part of la BAF's direct actions involve going out to meet people. It allows us to chat, share, and in a way, put faces and voices to ideas on a flyer or information found online. We are often present at music gigs, activist events, and neighborhood forums. And we never cease to be amazed at how quickly and comfortably people stop by to talk and open up to us, sometimes in an intimate way. For example, as a nurse and advocate for respectful gynecologic and obstetric practices, I've had a few discussions about gynecologic abuse while tabling in a corner of, say, a concert hall. Easily enough, people put their trust in us because they suppose la BAF, as feminist, is a "safe space." Even though this inference is not exactly correct, it sets people at ease. And it helps them to dare to go through the door of our library.

Doing outreach outside la BAF allows us to be better understood and more widely known, but allows us to grow our space and ourselves as well. For instance, we've ended up exchanging contact information with people we didn't know beforehand because they're interested in holding their own events at Au Chat Noir, such as popular education conferences, or *conférences gesticulées* in French—a popular education technique that's half stand-up comedy and half conference—film screenings, and *arpentages*—another popular education technique that consists of ripping a book into parts, then each participant has to read the pages they took on their own, and finally the group reconvenes to share each person's takeaway from their reading, "rebuilding" the torn book through the words and experiences of the eight or ten people who read some of its contents. We also gather ideas for new books to buy, zines on underrepresented topics, and new types of support groups. Meeting outside la BAF is a profoundly enriching experience, equally crucial to the life of the library as the actual space.

## TO BE OR NOT TO BE A SAFE SPACE

An important thing to know about la BAF is that it's not a safe space.[3] This fact may seem surprising or even shocking because, from a feminist cultural perspective, safety in general and safe spaces in particular have been central demands. So

---

3. This section was written by Éris.

how could this be?

To understand why our anarcha-feminist library isn't a safe space, we first have to understand what a safe space is (or rather, would be). A safe space is a place, actual or virtual (online groups or forums can be deemed "safe," for example), in which marginalized people are not at risk of violence or discrimination. Safe spaces are framed using affirmative ("LGBTQI+ people are welcome") or negative ("no racism, ableism, homophobia, transphobia ... allowed") language, frequently doubled up with regulatory means (moderators and mediators, "safety teams," or people in charge of intervening when somebody seems to disrespect the frame, often by kicking them out and taking care of the person who may have been hurt).

Safety, however, is itself a problematic concept.

First off, there is never any way to ensure 100 percent safety. It's all just harm reduction. Presenting a space as "safe" might actually make it *less* safe because if people walk in expecting to be shielded from any and all harm (each carrying their own sense of safety and own vulnerabilities based on their personal history), they are defenseless—and even more at risk from harm.

Second, we typically focus on what we want to be safe *from*; violence, discrimination, and so on, are experiences we seek to avoid. What if we instead asked ourselves, What are we safe *to*? Indeed, anarcha-feminist spaces—or any militant or "alternative" space, really—seek empowerment—that is, to enable people to do things that the larger/global society prevents or discourages. And while being safe *to* certainly requires a fair amount of safety *from*, there is a point where the two might contradict because ...

Third, in a society rife with discrimination of all kinds, demanding that an individual not engage in any of them is nearly, if not completely, impossible. As activists, we are (or should be) constantly learning, questioning our previous and current beliefs, listening to different views, and addressing issues as they arise. People who come into our spaces are not blank pages; they've soaked up a deeply unfair society. We can ask them—and each other—to put in the work, question their (often unconscious) prejudices, and listen to those people they may come to harm, but we can't ask that they know "everything" before they even join in our projects. In fact, a social justice culture that revolves around the usage of certain words and presents certain issues as somehow definitive (as if marginalized people never disagree on language or strategy) is likely to generate "correctness anxiety," making individuals (especially young or new to the struggle) afraid to speak or act lest they offend someone. Such "safe" spaces are *not* accessible because the amount of knowledge needed to come in is deeply elitist. They are *not* empowering either if one has to constantly walk on eggshells.

And finally, contrary to "safety," what we need is resilience. We need to generate spaces, both social and actual, in which mistakes are gently remarked, trying is praised, and expressing one's discomfort is met with thankfulness and the knowledge that it'll allow us to grow. Resilience isn't about not being hurt in the first place; it's about recovering from hurt. A resilient space is not one in which people never fall; it is one in which falling is OK because there is no hard ground to seriously injure us, and there are comrades to help us get back up again.

La BAF is not a safe space. It is a space to relax, read, study, or otherwise chill in; a space that opens up onto the neighborhood, with large, colorful windows; a space that is free to attend, of course, and anyone can wander in or out. Obviously, we—the volunteer librarians—would intervene if anything disrespectful or harmful happened, but there is no way to make sure that such things won't happen. That's because, for starters, we are de facto a public place, and there are a certain number of people out there who are less than happy about anarchism, feminism, or even open libraries; we have no bulky security guard to throw petty fascists out by the collar.

We're also, so to speak, an intermediary place. La BAF aspires to be a threshold and hopefully a door: we want people to come in because of the pretty books and free cookies, stay because they feel comfortable, and come back because they want to share our struggles or support them. We are aware we fail, and will keep failing, at being a door. Books are frightening or at least intimidating to many, and our own ease with being around books could make us seem elitist. But this manner of acting as a door, an open way into the struggle, is constitutive of who we are.

Some people who walk into the library may have never met a trans person in their lives or someone who's openly queer. How could they be anything but ignorant of the ways trans people and queers have developed among themselves? Sure, we'll—gently—correct them when they use incorrect pronouns, or use outdated language about disabilities (Is there even a language that disabled people among ourselves agree on?) or race (the same question applies). Yet *it will happen.*

People *will* use improper language. People *will* ask improper questions or make less-than-informed comments. They will. They just will. And we'll do our best to share what little we know with them.

We'll try to be *as safe a space as possible*. But we can't be a safe space. And between us, we think safe spaces simply don't exist.

Which, you know, is probably a good thing. Only from places where uncertainty and discomfort remain can we meet with people unlike ourselves, and share and learn from each other to build a world more resilient and kind.

## ON DOING NOTHING, AND ALL THE WORK IT ENTAILS

And there we stand on the threshold, the anarcha-feminist librarians.[4] It is peculiar indeed to act the part. Sometimes the best thing to do is nothing at all. Strangely, this may take more work than you would expect.

This may seem a little weird at first. We organize because we want to do things after all—usually a whole lot of things. But one of our goals at the library is to create (a) space for others. A space where people can come to explore, experiment, and enjoy; where they're free to do their own things and be their own selves. So sometimes what we need to do is nothing. Move back and open up some space for others to breathe.

Is it worth it? YES! When at last you sit back, sip some tea, and look at people doing their own cool stuff in the space you helped create, it can make your heart swell with pride. And sometimes they will even want to do things with you too! How

---

4. This section was written by Tom.

cool. But it's a lot of work to get there!

Because just doing nothing is not enough. You need to set up the stage a little, do some prep work. There are a lot of things to do before you can do nothing at last!

First, of course, you have to make people want to come to your place.

So you probably need to do some cool things of your own, you know, to jump-start things a little. To set a tone.

And you need to keep at it. Be open and reliable. Even when you do a screening of this cool movie, and the room is half empty. Or when you open the library for the afternoon, and nobody shows up ... three times in a row. Persist! If you do things that you enjoy anyway, they will always be a success. Even if it's just you and a few friends.

And advertise of course. If people don't know about you, all the doing nothing in the world will not amount to anything. Social networks are good for that, but you need to be OK with taking part in the system, so ... your call! Reach outward. Maybe there are alternatives, such as local mailing lists. Go see other people who do stuff you like and talk to them. Have some flyers in your bag and give them away.

Then you want people to stay.

Try to make things cozy. Have some nice places to sit, eat, and dream. Label food or keep the packaging around so that people can check what they can eat on their own. When it's cold, bring blankets and spread them around the space liberally.

Make tools available. Make it clear it is possible to do things, that this place is a space to express oneself. Offer inspiration. You want to encourage people to do things by themselves.

Try to provide clear means of guidance about what is possible and how things work. With drawings, not just words, if possible. You don't want people to depend on you to explain everything but instead to get used to doing things by themselves and running the place with you.

If people always have the same question, it could be a sign that something is missing. Can you supply them with the means to figure it out by themselves next time?

Take care of people. Reduce their mental load. Empower them to make decisions.

You also need to be there, of course. Open the place. Tidy up a little. Bring some sort of food (important!) and brew a pot of tea (*extra* important!). And since you're running a library, choose a good book to read—but not too good, since you won't have time to read it anyway.

So the place is set, the tea is hot, and you're starting to think that maybe, just maybe, for this once you will have some time to read this damn book ... and that's when they come in.

Now is not quite the time to do nothing yet!

Your job is now to make them cross not only the threshold from outside to inside but also from outsider to insider.

Ask questions and let them give the answers. Good starting questions are, "Did you come for the library?"—usually an easy one—and "Do you want a tour, or do you prefer to browse?" Let them decide how much space they want. Don't overload them. Let them breathe. Let them lead the pace.

Try to tell them, or better yet show them, that this is a place for people to do things, and so they can too. If the place is set so it's obvious, even better.

Once they're satisfied, let them know you're available if

they need help. And make sure you're available if they need it.

You want to make this place and moment theirs as much as yours.

If you've been good enough, they may even start doing cool stuff on their own. Don't be disappointed if they don't, though. Most people may not be up to it, and that's OK. But that can only happen if you're not already taking the space.

So now, at long last, is a good time do nothing! Serve some tea (you did remember to brew some tea, right?), look at your book (just look at it, don't read it; remember, be available!). Let them own the place.

And sometimes, just sometimes, they will come back to you and your space with a fire in their eyes and a head full of plans.

And everything becomes possible again.

❉  ❉  ❉

La Bibliothèque Anarcha-Féministe de Toulouse is a de facto association based in Toulouse. It is an open, self-organized library that tries to make theory, fiction, art books, comics, and zines accessible to the greatest number of people. The space also runs and participates in a number of varied cultural and activist events. You can reach Bibliothèque Anarcha-Féministe by email at bibli_afem@riseup.net or on Instagram @biblianarchafeministe.

# UNSANCTIONED SANCTUARIES: A CROSS-CONTINENTAL EXCHANGE

/

LIBERTIE VALANCE
AND XELA DE LA X

**Libertie:** So it feels funny introducing myself since I already know you, but because there are people listening in, here goes! I'm a nonbinary trans woman in my late thirties living in Southern Appalachia on Cherokee land. I've been involved in anarchist organizing since the late 1990s and early aughts, mostly in the South, and since 2008, I've been part of Firestorm, a queer anarchist feminist collective in Asheville, North Carolina. For the last seven years, our focus has been on running a radical bookstore where we also host events and provide accessible community resources.

**Xela:** I'm really blessed to have finally met you in person at the Institute for Advanced Troublemaking's summer camp class of 2019. Firestorm has shown support to our projects and various spaces throughout the years, and we are super grateful for that. Our collective is eleven years old now. We are unapologetically detribalized feminist anarchists, and run Casa C.O.A.T.L. aka The Shed, an autonomous anarcho-feminist space on occupied Tongvaland, and run by members of the OVAS—One Very Angry Squad, which was previously called the Ovarian Psycos cycling brigade. Growing in our analysis, solidifying our politics, and taking up space beyond the bicycle has become our primary focus as it allows us the opportunity to create the world we are fighting for, at least here for a moment, while we are still alive.

**Libertie:** Can you tell me a little bit more about Casa C.O.A.T.L.?

**Xela:** This is our third autonomous community-based space in Boyle Heights, a neighborhood in Los Angeles. The last two spaces were generally open to just about anybody, and many organizing circles formed out of the first space, La Conxa. We had nonstop community events and various organizing projects, including tenant defense, KYR [know your role] workshops, and study circles, punk/hip-hop shows, movie nights, open mics, and fundraisers toward endless causes, funerals, and solidarity efforts. The second La Conxa continued in this we'll-rest-when-we're-dead type of urgency. It was exhausting and clearly not sustainable.

At the new location, Casa C.O.A.T.L., we seemed to be heading in the same direction till COVID hit, and then we finally took a step back to reflect and check in with our hearts, spirits, bodies, and mentals. Plus the space, still rough, has taken us about two to three years now of ongoing rehab work. Yet the FTP [fomenting theory and praxis] community defense affinity group has had biweekly food and clothing distributions as well as a garden it started in the back. We now have a media room, where we are still experimenting with multimedia projects, and we also provide mutual aid and prisoner solidarity efforts with screen-printing projects. Lastly, we have a room for emergency housing specifically for femme, trans, and gender-nonconforming comrades who we know, should it be needed.

More than anything, this space is significantly different than the other two locations we've had mostly because our politics have shifted from mass organizing to now prioritizing our own needs and practicing being more intentional about building intimate relationships as we rebuild our ability to trust. Our last space was heavily attacked by authoritarians, which sadly included individuals we once organized shoulder to shoulder with under the now-defunct Defend Boyle Heights Coalition. The attacks have left scars, but along with the pandemic, the course of events forced us to insulate ourselves, allowing us to reevaluate and reimagine a sort of sanctuary or cocoon from which we can now explore our individual passions and interests. We've been cementing our politics, our boundaries, and collective care as we continue building on our skills while deepening our commitment and capacity. Ultimately our goal for our current space, Casa C.O.A.T.L. aka The Shed, is to shed all the ways we were burning ourselves out and focus our energies on multimedia, anarchist, antiauthoritarian, and femme of Indigenous descent propaganda.

**Libertie:** It's beautiful that you've created the spaces you need for each step of your collective journey. I guess I should share more about our physical space, since that's something we have in common! At the time of this conversation [in 2022], Firestorm is in its second location, a retail storefront in the commercial corridor of a residential neighborhood. We started off running a different kind of space downtown—a café, because that's what we had experience with. None of us had worked in bookstores. When we left downtown, it was an opportunity to grow into something new, and we picked a space we thought would be good for books.

Our collective first heard about y'all [the OVAS] in 2017. We screened the documentary film *Ovarian Psycos* about your activities in East LA and thought you were the dreamiest, coolest, most badass anarcha-feminists in the entire world. So when you and I met in 2019 at the Institute for Advanced

Troublemaking, I was already a fan!

**Xela:** Oh, that's so sweet. Thank you, but really we, or I should say I, don't know what the fuck I'm doing. I, like most folks, am just trying to figure shit out, print, love myself, and fuck shit up on my bicycle when I can.

**Libertie:** Bikes are such a cool starting point for a collective. I mean, I've heard about radical spaces that started with a study group or house shows, but it's really unique to begin as a bike crew. Anarcha-feminists on bikes reminds me of the film *Born in Flames* from the 1980s, which starts with a women's bike gang doing street interventions, like confronting patriarchal men and responding to assaults. Can you tell me more about how y'all got started?

**Xela:** So a couple of things happened at the same time. As is still the case today unfortunately, femmes of all ages are disappearing everywhere, including back-to-back instances of femmes murdered in our communities specifically, generating the desire to do something other than be fearful. And not wanting to instill fear in my daughter, not wanting to normalize misogyny or femicide but instead to reclaim our collective strength and ride at night, and intentionally take up the road, streets, corners, parks, and hills—all the locations where femmes had been killed—for the purpose of becoming a force to kill patriarchy, seemed more therapeutic and healing to us than lighting a candle at a vigil ever would.

In February 2010, I took my daughter to pick out a bicycle for her birthday, and she picked out a black one with orange and red flames, and the man working at the bike shop kept telling us that we were in the wrong section of the bike store and the "girls' bikes" were on the other side. I exchanged some words about how silly the idea of gendering a fucking bicycle was, and proceeded to demand that he either charge me for the bicycle that my daughter wanted or we would just take it and call it his gift to her. He shut the fuck up real quick; we paid and left the store content with my daughter's bicycle.

I taught her how to ride it right away and was struck by her fearlessness to be honest. And we began riding together weekly and talking about how legit it would be to start a crew. She recommended the name Fire Riders. Aw! But then we both really fell in love with the idea of playing with the *psyco* and *cycle* phonetics of it all. And then my car broke down soon after that, and one day on my way home from work on my bicycle, cars where literally at a standstill and everybody driving a car was visibly pissed because the streetlights had stopped working and so I remember maneuvering through all of that congested traffic feeling like, fuck yeah, on my bicycle I may just be unstoppable—at least as it relates to traffic.

**Libertie:** That's fantastic! You've been an anarchist and feminist for a long time. It sounded like maybe you got started in the punk scene, is that right?

**Xela:** I was an angry kid. I had a lot of rage and frustration, and punk spoke to that, but what was really awesome and unexpected were the groups and collectives with zines and mutual aid projects at the shows that redirected my rage in a way that gave more context and the possibility to create some dope shit with, whether that was music or collectives or other community projects, and build with folks who also understood and were down to make something beautiful out of the ugliness we live in. Then the Zapatista uprising sprouted a new movement here on the Eastside, reconnecting us to our roots, but with a much more political foundation and motivation that went beyond the aesthetics of our culture, really calling us to examine our place in history, our ties to the land, and ignite collective efforts in that spirit of Indigenous rebellion. The work with the PSYCOS has very much been influenced by my first collective, Cihuatl Tonali, identifying as urban Indigenous femmes, but many of us had come from punk shit. Just being angry knuckleheads, and for a fact at least back then, we identified hard core as Brown feminists of Indigenous descent and still anarchist. Made for this shit. To fuck shit up and smash the state. But maybe just a little different like, fuck the state. Create a world without asking anyone's permission.

**Libertie:** The Zapatistas have always embodied such incredible Indigenous feminist politics, it makes sense that they would be an entry point for your radicalization. I'm a few years behind you, so I got into anarchism in the late 1990s and then really started to understand myself as being part of a movement after the Battle of Seattle. That trajectory of global resistance owed an enormous debt to the Zapatistas.

I identified as a feminist before I was an anarchist. Growing up in a rural part of the South, being a feminist was the first "radical" identity I embraced. As a kid, I didn't really know anyone who claimed feminism, so it seemed sort of edgy. It's not like there weren't feminists in Southern Appalachia. I grew up not that far from bell hooks, but nobody told me about bell hooks. Instead I knew about Dolly Parton, who I idolized as a kid. It's funny that for liberal feminists, Dolly is a sort of icon, even though she won't even use the f-word. As a young adult, I started getting really excited about feminisms that were more aggressive and less interested in the success of middle- and upper-class white women.

**Xela:** You telling me about how you grew up reminds me that it's also super important that a lot of us here on the Eastside grew up under a lot of religious dogma, the omnipotent patriarchy of *god*, and for example, myself living under those conditions, the violence of subjugation. A lot of us in some form or another get pressed into submission, surrendering our power, bodies, desires, and dreams, under threat of punishment by god, the criticisms of society, and/ or the disownment of our fathers and/or brothers, and by extension the authority of our mothers perpetuating that—at least that was what I lived. Anywhere, any space that's created that is *not* that, spaces like Firestorm, for instance, or like here on the Eastside, are crucial to us throwing off that submission and figuring out what we want for ourselves. Besides us here in occupied Tongvaland, there's the Eastside Café, an autonomous community space; Corazón Del Pueblo, a collective, volunteer-run cultural center; and today, Memories of El Monte, a QTPOC community arts and mutual aid space. These spaces need to multiply and exist everywhere. Tell me what inspired y'all and how Firestorm got started.

**Libertie:** I was one of the folks who started the Firestorm Collective back in 2008. We understood ourselves as feminists and anarchists, but in the beginning we didn't really put those labels on our project because we weren't sure how people would respond. So we were organizing as anarchists, but we didn't tell our community for the first year. Later we learned that it was really important to be honest about who we were and that people would actually be excited to support an explicitly radical space. That's the first big thing I remember being wrong about. The first of many!

**Xela:** I hear that. We had similar misgivings about how to identify likely cuz of our inexperience, and just being happy that other femmes wanted to come ride bicycles in these streets at night to bark at the car when a man would drive by whistling or join us when we stopped at the detention centers to rage out "Fuck the police!" I assumed everybody coming out to the rides would clearly have to be feminist and anarchist, or at the very least would be bound to become one soon enough.

It seems that whether because we're poor, Brown, or rowdy, and zero fucks given, automatically our organizing efforts are suspect or underestimated and undermined. We can often internalize that shit and even undermine ourselves. I often feel I'm not doing enough or not doing it the "right way," but I have to catch myself and stop that cop in my head bullshit cuz really what the fuck is that? The "right way" according to whom? Doing enough as measured by what standard?

I was asked recently by an old friend, when was I going to grow up and go do something real with my life. He said,

"Like being a professor, get a career. You're too old for this."
Ha! And that's just it. If what we do is a joke, then fuck it,
I'd rather laugh. Ha! I'd rather play. I'd rather create space
with my homegrrrls where we can live and love and exist on
our terms, and plus if "professionalized" hetero cis men are
irritated with what our collective is doing or more specifically
what I'm doing with my life, then for a fact I'm on my chosen
path.

**Libertie:** I really admire that! When people ask you what it
means that you're an anarchist feminist project, what do you
tell them?

**Xela:** We are the squad you've been warned about. The
cautionary tale for all who struggle for a better world and are
actively organizing. To be feminist is to be vigilant about power
hierarchies that we may be re-creating in our interpersonal
relationships and within our own political analysis even—and
so be able to reflect on our own shit and be intentional about
destroying those hierarchical leanings within ourselves first.
And feminist because for the last five-hundred-plus years on
stolen land, we've been under patriarchy, particularly of the
white, cis, hetero variety, and that shit gotta go. Anarchist cuz
I will not obey. I refuse to willingly concede control of my life
or body—not to the state, not to a "god," not to a man. And
anarchists cuz we get a lot more done by ourselves or with
others who care beyond consumption and/or party lines.

**Libertie:** That's an incredible answer. I'm writing it down!
(*laughs.*) Our attachment to anarcha-feminism is similarly

rooted in what we've experienced and the ways that we choose to come together as a collective.

Sometimes people are like, "Oh, so is every book in your store about anarchism?" And of course the answer is "no." We have a lot of titles by anarchists, but it's not our catalog that makes our project anarchist, it's us. Our feminism is informed by the experience of misogyny and patriarchal violence. We want to create a space together that breaks away from all of that—prioritizing empowerment, consent, and accountability. And as a cooperative, we're also working to confront and dismantle the toxic shit that goes along with workplace culture.

I remember when we first started, there were people in our community who were pretty hostile toward us because they thought we were just reproducing capitalism or recuperating anarchism by running a business. And that bummed us out, but we also understood the concern. Ultimately, I think we had to win people's respect by consistently showing up and being solid comrades. It probably helps that we kept getting into fights with the city. (*laughs.*) When we were still in our first location, which was downtown, we helped lead a campaign against a business improvement district that would have created a private police force controlled by property owners. (We won that fight!) In recent years, we've worked with the Steady Collective, a harm reduction program that distributes Naloxone and clean injection supplies primarily to folks on the street. Folks who are disproportionately queer and trans.

In our community, drug users and unhoused folks are on the receiving end of a lot of abuse because they detract from a vision of Asheville as an upscale tourist playground. In 2018, the city tried to shut down the Steady Collective's syringe access program that was happening once a week in our space. It was kind of surreal because the zoning department actually claimed we weren't a real bookstore. I don't think anyone from the city even came in to see if we had books, they just drove by and saw homeless people, which in their estimation made us a homeless shelter—an illegal homeless one. So we got hit with a "notice of violation" threatening fines and potential prosecution if we didn't stop hosting harm reduction work. When we refused to comply, we received a lot of community support. At one point, we heard that the zoning department had to take its phones off the hook because so many pissed-off people were calling in. The fight consumed a year of our lives, but in the end we won. And we never stopped hosting the syringe access program, not for one day. But fights like that also wear you down.

I think that we're probably the most anarchist when we're navigating conflict or challenges within our collective. Those are the moments when we really have an opportunity to do something different, to unlearn the patterns of dysfunction and harm that we've experienced in other spaces. So we try to slow down and ask each other how we want to be treated, how we want to be cared for. Even when we're mad at each other!

**Xela:** Recently somebody mentioned that they try to stay away from conflict, right? And my initial response was, "I enjoy conflict!" But that was a lazy way of saying it doesn't bother me. I feel like in those moments of conflict, you can really understand each other at a different level. So if something bothered you or whatever, let's unpack that further and then I can have a better understanding of where you're coming from, and hopefully you have a better understanding of where I'm coming from. I think we've been so conditioned to center our hurt feelings—and they matter, sure—but ultimately, where does the relationship that we've built for, say, ten years matter? Or does it even matter?

**Libertie:** This is something that shows up for us. Conflict avoidance can be a product of white supremacy culture, and while it's not only white people who replicate white supremacy, for us, as a majority-white collective, we've really struggled with this dynamic. Many of us were raised not talking through conflicts or being told that women should keep their voices down. But if we're going to have healthy relationships, we have to be less fragile and willing to have conflicts.

**Xela:** Our collective is primarily Brown, and we've been indoctrinated to not stir anything up, or keep our voices low or just swallow it, even at the detriment of our continued discomfort. I see it still in organizing spaces like ours. I've been told, continuously, that it's my tone, so I've experimented with that. I've tried to sing it. I'll try to say it sweetly. But it doesn't matter. It's the point that I'm speaking, even if I say, "Come on, we're sisters. If my tone was this way, if I curse this way, I wasn't cursing you." I think it goes back to how we're stuck in carceral dynamics, even the surveillance of how we speak. One time I started putting duct tape around my mouth, so that I wouldn't interrupt. But then it became an issue of, "Xela, we didn't like the way you rolled your eyes or how you looked at us." So then I'm sort of stuck with surveillance of how I'm processing things. Yet I'm a human being; I can't show up with a poker face.

And then there are relationships where the conflict has kind of solidified our friendship. In the times where I know their heart, I'm not going to take it personally. I think that's really important, knowing each other's heart, if that makes any sense. For example, I do a lot of the labor in our space and am hardly online, so there's no reason to feel like I am trying to gain clout! So I think that my actions should speak to the fact that I'm committed to this work in this way. We need to really be sitting with and reflecting on each other's motivations, because you know I'm not above petty jealousies! You know what I'm saying? I'm not above all kinds of fucking behaviors. So we should really sit down and reflect on our actions, and our motivations behind those actions. It's also really important to understand that nobody is fucking perfect, but can we experiment further on how to hold space for each other in a compassionate way? Because clearly, we're not each other's enemy. Regardless of whether you share the same geographic or cultural background, we share at least affinity in terms of our politics—antiauthoritarian or anarchist if you want to call it that.

It makes me think about mutual aid and how I've seen where everybody knows what to do to tangibly share resources, whether food or clothes. And I wonder about mutual aid in terms of emotional mutual aid. Where it's actually much more difficult because you have to be in your feelings. It's less physical labor; I'm not having to access a car to go pick up the food. I just have to access my emotions and be mutually reciprocal with the other person and understand that we all fuck up. I think that takes priority with the folks who we call comrades, even with family. I think that takes precedence over the tangible sharing of the resources.

**Libertie:** That's really insightful. I like the idea of emotional mutual aid. I'm curious if you have any norms or practices that support communication within your collective? How do y'all manage relationships?

**Xela:** Well, back in the day, we used to do a very tankie type of practice: crit self-crit. (*laughs.*) Then, instead, we tried to do what's called Spinoza's roses: Where do we have flowers and where do we have thorns? But one of the things that I saw happening a lot was this need to pathologize each other. That's kind of fucked up, because that's why the collective has the word *psycho* in it, meaning, "Yeah, the world is crazy." If what I'm doing is seen as crazy, we're already pathologized. So I didn't understand the need to pathologize ourselves further. It felt like surveillance culture and the easy way out of things. So nowadays, with the collective members who we have currently, we just talk it out if there's an issue.

One collective I was a part of before had an interesting practice: whenever there was discord, or if there was conflict between two folks, we had two options. You could box it out— some kind of jujitsu domination, or for people who weren't into that, you could give the gift of forgiveness, or the gift of just simply being present for each other to be able to discuss it further. But these days what we're trying to do is before every meeting, have a real honest check-in, a check-in of the heart, not just how your day is or how your week has been going.

**Libertie:** And what do you think makes that work? Do you rely on people who aren't part of the collective to support communication when there's conflict?

**Xela:** No, if the conflict is between two people, we have a member who does her best at hearing both sides. Nobody officially made her the mediator, but she does it and just has skills. But sadly we did lose a member recently who needed space because they just didn't have capacity, emotional capacity, to try to resolve things, and I wish them the best. Ultimately that is a personal decision. You can't force anybody to make the space so that together we can figure it out.

**Libertie:** It's hard doing this under capitalism because there's so many limitations placed on people's ability to show up.

**Xela:** Yeah, but one of the things that we did even back then was have a hard agreement that whatever gets shared, should never be weaponized or put in a pocket for later. How do you all do it?

**Libertie:** I agree that it's easier to navigate relationships when you really know someone; you kind of know their context and story. A lot of times, when somebody doesn't show up in a good way, there's something going on for them. So we try to make a lot of space to talk about what's going on for us outside our work together. We've also experimented with different ways of creating space for relationship building.

For instance, we were doing a thing where every month,

every member of our collective would sit down with every other member for one hour and just have a conversation. It didn't have to be about the bookstore or a project we were working on together. It could be about anything—maybe something going on in your personal life. The hope was that we could understand where each other were coming from and have that baseline of empathy for when we step on each other's toes. Then maybe we get upset with each other, but we're able to temper that with knowledge and understanding of what's going on. And we know some dynamics that we can fall into, things to be careful about.

In terms of actual conflicts, we used to do a lot of work with outside mediators. Around the time of Occupy in 2012, we had several connections in the community to people who were really good at facilitating difficult conversations, and they could come in and help everyone feel heard while uncovering things that weren't immediately obvious to the rest of us.

We haven't really had those relationships in the last few years, so we've approached conflict similarly to what you were describing: we create space in meetings to bring it out and give it room. We try to honor the conflict rather than treat it as irrelevant or act like it should be dealt with outside collective space. We've also tried to learn about each other's communication and work styles. There's an exercise we do where we all answer a series of questions, things like "What do you need when you're stressed out?" and "What are your most closely held values?" Then we talk through our answers, and it starts to form a sort of map of how we work together. And we can give each other explicit instructions, like "Here's the thing that I really do or don't want you to do for me when

I'm struggling."

**Xela:** That's beautiful.

**Libertie:** It's been useful. It also means that when a new person starts working with us, we can have them answer the same questions, but then also share all the answers that we've previously written out. I think it's nice for new people. So they'll know that if I'm really cranky, I probably need to eat food. (*laughs.*)

**Xela:** Classic me too! It makes me think of back in the day, when we were like thirteen deep, we used to have a thing every season where we would randomly pick each other's names from a hat and then that person was going to be your best friend for the season. You had to hang out with each other and figure each other out and share with each other.

**Libertie:** Something I'm hearing from you, that I know is true for us as well, is this idea of experimentation. It's clear that both of our collectives have never settled on one thing, right? We keep trying new things, and I think that's really very anarcha-feminist of us! We just keep coming back to this question of how we care for our relationships and create new organic patterns. It's never about finding the perfect thing or following a party line. It's about new experimental forms.

**Xela:** Absolutely. For example, our other spaces always had principles of unity. Then we changed to principles of solidarity, and then it was, like, principles of war [when we were attacked by tankies]. But then, finally, we were like fuck principles! Let's understand our personal constitution. What are the agreements that I make? Our body is our first territorial defense, right? And so understanding that our body was our first territory, then what are my personal principles, my personal values, my constitution? What does that look like? It's important to understand our own personal constitution because then we can create agreement for the space. And then when we collaborate with folks, they have the option to be in alignment with that or not. The idea of boundaries is so intangible, like when a person says, "You crossed my boundaries" or "You're not respecting my boundaries." How would I know, unless I know your personal constitution? That's what fortifies each of us individually, understanding what our boundaries materially and tangibly look like, right? So that's one thing that we've been practicing, and it's been interesting because it's been a harder task to think about our own boundaries in this way. To put actual sentiments and words and feelings to that, as opposed to principles for the space, which is theoretical.

**Libertie:** That sounds similar to our experience. Our collective is negative on policies and rules that people need to follow. Instead we try to build a shared culture that changes as our needs change. Maybe that looks like generating a collectively written document, but we write statements and not contracts. Sometimes we end up sharing those statements publicly too—as a form of transparency or to help people understand what we're doing. Years ago, we wrote some collective agreements to guide our work together in meetings.

We have a lot of meetings! And the agreements included things like respecting each other's time. But what does respecting someone's time actually mean? It's so culturally specific. So whenever a new person joins our collective, we have to look at the agreements again and revise them. Which is good because it also gives us a chance to ask ourselves if our agreements still reflect the culture we're striving for. They have to stay fluid because relationships are fluid.

Maybe we could also talk a little bit about the mistakes we've grown from, because some of those mistakes at Firestorm were related to our feminism, and I know y'all struggled with your identity and original name, Ovarian Psycos.

**Xela:** The name was speaking initially to the immediate issues of those in the collective, which originally was just me and my daughter. As our collective grew, we got a lot of heat on a variety of issues. Like we were not real cyclists cuz we didn't wear the right clothing nor were we posting constant clocking in of our miles, so who cares? We can't afford your fancy gear, jerks! Or, for example, why not let men ride? And we were like, well, fuck it. Men can hold the water for us, if they want. Ha! Maybe some people thought we were really arrogant, but nah, nah, this collective is for us women. So we doubled down, but then we got schooled appropriately on the fact that not all women have ovaries.

**Libertie:** Was that feedback from your local community or strangers on the internet?

**Xela:** On the internet, but even to our faces. Our politics were still in development, but we recognized the error in equating women with ovaries, so now we go by OVAS.

**Libertie:** I think it's great that after hearing how your shit was landing for people with different experiences, you wanted to change it up, to make it clear that you were in solidarity with trans folks.

Firestorm had some experiences that were maybe a little similar. I think you can't run a public project and not get called on some shit. And sometimes maybe you disagree with the call, but you still learn something. Early in Firestorm's history, our collective didn't describe itself as queer or trans. We brought those identities with us, but it wasn't the basis of our organizing. So at some point, in maybe 2009, we got into conflict with a radical trans crew in our town. I think these folks didn't understand us to be part of their community, and they approached us with the same suspicion that queer and trans people often approach straight spaces. They were upset because we booked an event with an artist who we didn't know had played the Michigan Womyn's Music Festival.

**Xela:** That was a TERF festival, right?

**Libertie:** Yeah. But I honestly didn't know anything about it at the time. So we booked this feminist musician Bitch, who was on Ani DiFranco's record label, and a couple days before the show we found out that people were tearing down and defacing our flyers. Asheville is a small town, so we figured out who was doing it, and asked them to sit down and talk to us. By the time we sat down together, this group of mostly trans women was really pissed at us because we hadn't canceled the show. And we were pretty unhappy with them for not coming to us directly, you know, for not extending us the opportunity to hear them and act in solidarity without having our arms twisted. In the end, we went back to the artist and made a proposition: we wouldn't cancel the show on the condition that they participate in a community conversation about trans exclusion and be accountable to their involvement in MichFest.

**Xela:** At the very least have a goddamn conversation. Yes, yes.

**Libertie:** Right. Well it was short notice, but it seemed reasonable. Bitch decided not to play the show, so there wasn't a public conversation, but it was still a big lesson for our collective. We realized that we had a responsibility to be more careful with the content that we platformed, and I think some of us also started thinking about how we needed to better communicate who we were to our community, because for me the hardest part of it was not being recognized by other trans people.

**Xela:** Yeah, I think that's important. That's why we have been open about reflecting on the terms being used. Like, if our shit sounds TERFy, then fuck that noise because that's *not* what we are about. And because patriarchy affects even men, even cis men, it affects everybody. It affects the whole damn world at the end of the day, like colonization affects the whole damn world.

But thank you for sharing what you all went through. It does matter. It all matters at the end of day, like being better humans to each other without centering humans over animals, plants, flowers, and all living creatures, and dead ones as well.

**Libertie:** We all need practice talking through difficult stuff. It's clear that most of us have experienced being silenced or not having our concerns taken seriously, and so we haven't developed the skills we need to communicate. Or we don't have a culture that supports effective communication. I think it's good when projects like the OVAS or Firestorm get a chance to build our skills, and maybe even model effective responses to conflict and harm.

When I think about feminism, one of the things I think about a lot is how we respond when people are experiencing harm. Within our collective over the years, we've had a lot of opportunities to confront toxic behavior and we made mistakes, especially early on. We didn't hold people accountable effectively and weren't really holding ourselves accountable. Then even when we started taking anti-oppression work seriously, we were slow to recognize how harm played out between queer and trans people. But I guess the thing that we did right is that we didn't give up, and when people criticized us—we didn't use that as an excuse to stop trying. Those experiences have been really foundational to my feminism.

The way you were talking about how much you give—and how much community spaces like Casa C.O.A.T.L. are giving—makes me think about how movement spaces are a type of feminist direct action. What I mean is that there's a tendency to gender the work that supports movements. The work of maintaining a space and caring for a community's physical needs, it's reproductive work, you know. It's the work of caring for our radical movements, and a lot of radical men don't want to do that work, or they do it and then move onto something more prestigious. I guess nobody is writing books about the nineteenth-century anarchists who cleaned the bathrooms in the Paris Commune! Chances are they were women.

❊   ❊   ❊

Firestorm can be found in real life at 1022 Haywood Road, its third and maybe final location in Asheville, or online at https://firestorm.coop.

Casa C.O.A.T.L. can be found in the for-real life at 2515 East Cesar E. Chavez Avenue, Boyle Heights, California, unless the building is sold, as it's actively on the market. OVAS is blessed to have shared spaces, labor, laughs, rage, and (psyco/cycle) paths with all who gave their energy and those who have supported all three iterations of our autonomous spaces/experiments in refusal. Xela can be found likely ripping out the floors, starting from the bottom, at another abandoned location near you.

# TARPS AND GOSSIP: EXISTING AS RESISTING

/

RAANI BEGUM

Nowadays, the grounds around McPherson library are quiet. Led by real estate profiteers and the city government, a combination of cold, constant encampment sweeps and an organized effort to drive away every community outreach to unhoused people has had a profound impact on Kensington. Still, unhoused drug users and sex workers remain. This Philadelphia neighborhood has had a culture of unhoused drug users and sex workers for over two centuries now. No wonder it is resilient.

Nightshade, a collective community space by and for outdoor and poor sex workers and drug users run jointly by Project SAFE and the Philadelphia Red Umbrella Alliance, was formed in 2016.[1] A proud member of Nightshade, I joined during my early sex working days sometime in 2017 and became a core organizer in 2020. After the 2020 lockdowns started, we shifted to gathering in open public spaces; the goal was both risk mitigation due to the pandemic and meeting people right where they were at, quite literally.

When we began those outdoor meetings, the park grounds were extremely lively and lived in by unhoused neighbors. People set up tents together, shared their resources, and became entangled with and looked out for each other. I want to be explicit here: drug use and sex work is a part of life for many living in Philadelphia. Nightshade is an extension of this culture. So people share tips and tricks on drug use,

---

1. For more on Project SAFE, a peer-based, grassroots harm reduction organization, see https://projectsafe.com/. For more on the Philadelphia Red Umbrella Alliance, an all-volunteer, sex-worker-run collective, see https://phillyrua.com/. *Editor's note*: It's a sweet coincidence that Nightshade is the name of two, albeit unrelated, collectives in this anthology (see "The Collective as a Crucial Form").

sex work, and raising money in myriad other ways, and accessing resources including shelter. Most people are queer and/or disabled, and many intersections of lived experiences converge at Nightshade.

When oppressed people openly claim a space, they are faced with hostility. Kensington is no different. Police presence is a constant. I have witnessed cops idly circle around repeatedly in their SUVs to inspire terror, stage violent arrests, bike up on people in droves, and kick sleeping people awake. The violence does not stop there. In response to decades of organizing against policing, diversion programs such as Police Assisted Diversion and Dawn Court, a postdiversion-ary program, extend "benevolent" carceral violence. These programs, a coalition between police, city government, and nonprofits, promise to put people through rehab and mental health treatment with the stipulation that participants must exit the drug and sex trades. Yet with no job or real housing opportunities, participants find themselves trapped in a cycle of poverty and incarceration. Then there is the issue of medical care. As the US government decreases the supply of pain medication, stimulants, and other lifesaving care, more people find themselves unable to hold onto what's necessary to survive capitalism. More people end up living on the street, revolving through various programs and jails, and the carceral system uses their visibility and plight to escalate conflict between housed and unhoused neighbors. Profiteers promise a "cleaner and safer neighborhood" to residents, and use this pledge to support violent encampment sweeps to pursue gentrification. These are the conditions in which Nightshade exists.

Still, every week a few housed sex workers open up space by laying down a poly tarp in our designated spot in a park. We come bearing a cartful of kits packed with harm reduction, safer sex, and first aid supplies. There is hot coffee and tea, and bottled water gets passed around. Sometimes we are able to bring clothes, shoes, donuts, pepper spray, coloring pages and pencils, knickknacks, and other small or portable items to exchange. We share bad dates sheets—pieces of paper with descriptions of clients who may have robbed, assaulted, or otherwise caused a sex worker grief. We ask for "bad date" and "bad [drug] batch" reports, emphasizing that we do not work with the police and take no identifying information from workers.

While we bring supplies and information, it is important to understand that Nightshade is not focused on direct service. We catch up with each other. Someone brings along a new member, and another person talks about considering rehab. We sit with each other on the tarp and color while discussing the poisoned street drug supply, swapping humorous sex working anecdotes, and telling each other about our hopes for our personal and collective futures. Sometimes people come to nap. There is no preassigned agenda. Every meeting is different from the last. And how could it not be? At the end of the day, Nightshade at its heart is just a time and place where a group of sex workers come to meet each other and exchange gossip. No two gossip sessions are alike.

When I sat down to write this piece, I wanted to extract some deeper organizing wisdom gained from our gatherings. The truth of the matter is, we are just some whores stubbornly carving out something in a space wrecked by unimaginable hostility. As sex workers and drug users, we are not seen as people able to manage ourselves and our lives. We are viewed as too stupid to care for ourselves, too airheaded to make our own decisions, too materialistic to organize ourselves, and too zombied out to defend ourselves. Institutional violence deems us as "not human," and this translates palpably in the ways we are treated.

Rather than being stymied by it, it gives our organizing more freedom. Unlike other organizing spaces, Nightshade is not goal oriented. It is instead oriented toward friendship and rest. Some of my favorite Nightshade memories are of people coming to nap. Not only do we build relational trust that allows napping to happen, but we model community naps and community rest. Then there are the gossip sessions. Because the conversation is easy and flowing, we can ask each other more in-depth questions about where our various perspectives are coming from and gently interrogate internalized stigma when it inevitably rears its head. Here, I learned that some of my friends enjoyed outdoor living and scrutinized my own preconceptions about unhoused people. I have also gotten to share the different ways I work and been able to support members when they wish to transition to different parts of the erotic labor industry. In this way, we cover vast terrains of politically deep conversations stretching from race in sex work, to overdose prevention sites and safe supply, to encampment organizing.

In this context, Nightshade is a protest too, week in and week out. On a sunny afternoon during the retelling of a boisterous joke, a librarian comes over to tell us we should not be serving food to unhoused people. We counter that we are just a group having a picnic with friends and family and successfully send him away. Other encounters do not always end so smoothly. On a quiet fall day, a cop comes over and wakes up one of our members from her nap, feigning concern over an overdose, despite our vehement protest. That day, while we were unable to stop a cop from enacting violence on our autonomy and breaching our space, we modeled what community self-defense and solidarity looks like. Abolishing the police is a deeply held value in Nightshade. To detractors of police abolition, sex workers in the open experiencing violence may be an excellent example of why we need police as protection. But we don't. We protect ourselves from hostile neighbors and the police. We prove to ourselves that a new world is possible.

Nightshade continues to survive as a space where we self-determine how we love and value each other. In foregrounding this space in camaraderie, we become conspiratorial. Here, neither collective care nor community defense feel aspirational. Rather, it is an easy thing we extend to each other. Under systems designed to eradicate our existence, we quietly create an oasis as a manifestation of a more collective future.

❖   ❖   ❖

Raani Begum, a queer, migrant, disabled, full-service sex worker, is a core organizer in Project SAFE and the Philadelphia Red Umbrella Alliance, and a member of Heaux History and Mad Ecologies. They also read, build, community, and write. Raani is interested in how topics of sentiment and propaganda, anarchist world-building, and global histories of sex work and drug use intersect. She comes from Pakistan and Myanmar, and leans on their migrant and sex working knowledge when community building. They accept all pronouns, including her name, in good faith. You can find Raani at raanibegum.com.

# BROWN GIRL RISE: HOW WE TAKE CARE OF OUR OWN

/

CLAIRE BARRERA

In winter and spring 2017, a group of adult women and nonbinary people, mostly Black and Brown, came together in Portland, Oregon. Some of us were the mothers of Black and Brown girls and femmes. Some of us were young Black adults who had once ourselves been Black girls and femmes growing up in Portland. And some of us were expert childcare workers and career healers. All of us, individually and in our friendships, were thinking about the difficulties facing young girls and nonbinary youths of the global majority growing up in a majority-white city with an egregious history of anti-Black and anti-Brown racism.

A feature of community-led, anarchist organizing is that we recognize a need or problem and respond, finding an organic solution from within. We know what is really happening from lived experience and we know what we need; we do not look to or trust the authority of the state to identify and address our concerns. As children, the adults who became the original Brown Girl Rise (BGR) collective had personally experienced dealing with white supremacy in Portland's schools, neighborhoods, medical settings, and more. The parents among us were learning how hard it was to find affinity spaces and culturally affirming education for our kids, particularly for Black girls and nonbinary youths, and noticing how our children suffered as a result of this lack. And many of us had worked in environments where youths were telling us what they needed: "I had just come out of working at [an Indigenous organization] and really seeing youths not have any understanding of their body, but also craving that education," founding member Allie shares. "We're failing our youths, and we wanted to create a space that was safer, and actually addressed the resilience of our communities as well as the histories and realities of violence, but also empower folks with understandings of the body and ways to find agency and sovereignty in their bodies."

So the question arose among us: How do we take care of our own? Could we offer our youths the space to build relationships with each other, the adults in their communities, and their cultures and ancestries? BGR was established to do just that.

## SISTERHOOD

Many of the people involved in BGR had histories of working in nonprofits or government agencies, and had been burned by the ways the state insinuated itself into every aspect of that work. BGR didn't want to re-create typical nonprofit models of youth service provision, and we continue to resist the pull of professionalization and the culture of white supremacy at every turn.

Dani, who had worked with neurodivergent youths in nonprofit settings prior to working with BGR, names how nonprofits expect a kind of false, authoritarian division between the service provider, youth "client," and family surrounding the youth. She says, "When I worked with youths in other organizations, it was really like, I'm there solely for the youths and I don't listen to the parents. The parents aren't a concern to me because having a relationship with the parents would jeopardize my relationship with the youths. Like it wouldn't serve them as well."

Dividing our personal and professional selves, including in care and educational professionals, is an effective tool to divide us from our communities, empathy, and shared humanity. It's also a missed opportunity for reciprocal healing; the person providing care loses the chance to be healed in return by the person receiving care. And as Gloria notes, "It's extractive, by the organization, when you're not getting the healing back in that process."

We knew that we wanted to break down the walls erected between us by those in power and instead build interdependence. To do that, sisterhood became central to the mission of BGR from the start. We understand *sisterhood* to mean a feminist expression of deeply committed relationships in which reciprocal care and mutuality are seen as the primary forms of resistance and generation. BGR made sure to provide programming that wrapped around the entire family unit, not just the young person involved. For instance, we held social events like movie nights and had gatherings just for parents to chat with each other while the youths had workshops. Or we met up at protests and performances so we could deepen relationships and create solidarity space.

Like an abuser, the state would see us isolated, unable to make the connections that would allow us and our youths to free ourselves and create new worlds. Women and nonbinary people of the global majority in particular are kept from collective wisdom and affinity spaces, expected to manage our grief and anger in private. Allie observes that "we're constantly having to hold ourselves and be good on our own, and have that kind of constriction in our bodies and spirits." But in BGR, "sisterhood means looking at our relationships and striving to decolonize them with each other, because so much of it has been internalized and lateral violence."

In *Joyful Militancy*, coauthors Nick Montgomery and carla bergman point to the way that

> non-nuclear kinship networks have been sustained in the face of state terrorism and incarceration, residential and boarding schools, and Empire's ongoing attempts to privatize and destroy non-nuclear kinship networks, extended families, and webs of relationships that include nonhuman kin. Nourishing and sustaining these communal forms of life throws into question some of the dominant ideas about ... [the] separation of activism or organizing from everyday life. They challenge the segregation of kids from the rest of the world (and from organizing and politics in particular) and the ways that elders are isolated and intergenerational connections are lost.[1]

As organizers, we want to cultivate solidarity between ourselves and between youths. Further, we want to nurture it between generations. We believe that kinship in the face of state violence is a radical affirmation of the value of our lives. We also see sisterhood as primary to achieving lasting and profound change, where we can resource each other outside the transactional and scarcity-oriented programs of the state.

Building intergenerational relationships and centering youth leadership is not always easy. BGR has frequently come up against the ageism that permeates our world. The parents in our organizing collective are all older than the other members who do the majority of the direct youth work.

---

1. Nick Montgomery and carla bergman, *Joyful Militancy: Building Thriving Resistance in Toxic Times* (Oakland, CA: AK Press, 2017), 10.

We've created a youth advisory board and hired a former program participant. Finding the line between mentorship and condescension, between youth empowerment and lack of support, is really difficult. On the one hand, youth collective members have called the adults in on behaviors like not taking their ideas as seriously or giving their voices equal space. On the other hand, our organization continues to grapple with our youth board and workers being at a different place in their learning and development. Youths often need more teaching, modeling, and logistical support because of the simple fact that they've had less practice in the world. A desire to empower our young people by giving them control of the organization has meant that at times, things aren't getting done or done well. And youths sometimes feel unsupported and lost in that dynamic. BGR continues to seek a balance that will avoid these pitfalls.

In our work with youths, the emphasis on kinship has meant that our programming activities concentrate on relationships between youths rather than between youths and adult/authority figures. Much time is spent in games and relationship-building activities. Opportunities for risk or pushing the learning edge (such as our annual campouts) allow youths to express vulnerability as well as turn to each other for support and creative solutions to problems, including social concerns. Addressing allyship by focusing workshops on different identities (that is, disabled folks, LGBTQIA+, Indigenous people, etc.) builds sisterhood as well; youths learn to value the self and others equally along with the skills to be in solidarity with the kids around them.

Practicing sisterhood has at moments been difficult when

organizers or families do not feel deserving of care, or experience vulnerability in relationships as unsafe. As communities impacted by injustice, many of us struggle with imposter syndrome. We've had organizers who had to leave because they weren't showing up to do the work, but they also weren't able to accept the support to address their needs and stay in our community. Trauma can make sustaining relationships incredibly hard.

But we've had success too. In 2020, both organizers and the families we worked with were deeply impacted economically and socially by the violence of the COVID-19 pandemic and ongoing racial genocide. Because we had spent three to four years building deep connection, we were able to quickly act in support of each other. Mutual aid was already a key component of how we worked. In spring 2020, our organization made regular calls to families and youths to check in on their well-being, and delivered thousands of dollars in mutual aid as well as food deliveries and care packages. Moreover, our organizing collective brought each other meals and groceries, fundraised for each other, met regularly online to process our feelings, and attended antiracist protests together in groups. We knew the ins and outs of each other's lives, and our focus on relationships meant that we had already normalized reciprocal care. Giving and receiving support was therefore easier than it would have been otherwise.

## FIERCE LOVE

At the level of the BGR organizing collective, the way we practiced sisterhood became synonymous with the term *fierce love*, which was coined a few years into our work and play together. As Dani defines it,

> Fierce love is loving people authentically and as they show up, and really loving people to the point where you allow them to be their full self around you and also to make that love a priority over everything else. I think in our work we are constantly dealing with deadlines and having to present to the world in a certain way to make the work that we're doing seem legitimate. And I think the way that we really fight against that is with fierce love. No deadline matters as much as the needs of people within this collective.

This emphasis on the fierceness of our love for each other is about a militant resistance to the ways that the culture of white supremacy constantly tries to worm its way into our work and relationships. For example, it continually promotes a state of urgency and crisis. Our collective members struggle with the feeling all the time that we're not doing enough, and what we are doing isn't happening fast enough. Funders and other institutions push this value on us further with inflexible deadlines and persistent demands on our work. But we push back by "moving at the pace of trust," as Ashnie, a parent and BGR auntie, says, adding,

The pace at which we're growing is at the pace of trust, which is of course slower. So I think one of the things that is different for us as an organization is, on the one hand, we've achieved so much, and on the other hand, *if* we weren't, you know, bothering with this fierce love thing and caring about each other, we would move at a pace that would have accomplished things that culturally look successful. But we've redefined what success looks like with the value of fierce love at the center.

We have worked as a collective to turn down opportunities that overburden us and pivot our programming to adjust to reasonable workloads for the leadership team. We don't wish to replicate the values that created the problem in the first place.

Fierce love has also come to mean a commitment to holding each other accountable even as we give each other care and understanding. In fact, these two things go hand in hand. As Dani puts it,

> Accountability is a big part of fierce love. The way that we hold each other accountable is to really remind each other of our inherent goodness. Anytime I'm reminded, anytime somebody calls me in, you know, it's always to remind me that I can treat myself better or that what I'm doing is not the way I have to be doing it. I have the capacity to make changes that are good for myself and good for my community as a whole.

This is often the way accountability has shown up in our collective: to address the ways that shame and internalized oppression have impacted our ability to be present in our work. Typically when there is an issue, such as someone not following through on a commitment or acting in an oppressive way toward others, the person is addressed directly. But in addition to being told honestly about the impact of their behavior, they are listened to as well as offered compassion, resources, and support in making changes. We understand that people's behaviors do not exist in a vacuum and that change is only possible if the root causes are addressed collectively. It may be that something needs to change in the structure of our work as much as the individual needs to grow personally. As Grace underscores, "Accountability for us was never a set of protocols, and always a matter of trying to love each other and our community more deeply, more radically."

Fierce love is sometimes unsuccessful when fear of conflict and a sense of danger get in the way. As mentioned before, we each struggle with histories of trauma and marginalization. Conflict has been incredibly harmful for many of us in the past. Sometimes collective members have avoided speaking their truths because of this. At other times, some of us have been defensive and unreceptive to being called in, even with love. We experience a critique of behavior as a judgment on who we are as people, and this can cause intense anxiety.

A powerful example of successful fierce love in action, though, occurred in late summer 2020. Two of our young, Black coordinators, Grace and Dani, approached the collective to let us know the ways that ageism and anti-Black oppression were impacting them and our programming at large. They shared the ways that they had felt marginalized and shut down, particularly by non-Black and older organizers. Their concerns were taken seriously and addressed via changes in personal behaviors as well as organizational practices. We poured further care into each other rather than pulling away or engaging in performative change.

Grace shares that

> what was really transformative for me in my role at BGR in terms of accountability was that it was never like "Grace, this wasn't right" or "Grace, where is this thing that you committed to doing?" It was always a question of, "What kind of connection do you need to feel supported in doing this specific thing?" or "What comes up in your physical body when you are doing this thing?" Always trying to work with people as human beings with urgent social, emotional spiritual needs and *not* as productivity machines.

This means that fierce love is about process over product in our organizing, including creating space for intergenerational vulnerability. "We as adult facilitators," explains Grace,

> were holding space for young people dealing with racism, homophobia, and sexism in their everyday lives and trying to foster solidarity. Doing that facilitation authentically meant sharing our own experiences and opening up about what we do to move through those spaces with wholeness—always recognizing that we are part of a continuum of Black and Brown femme

experiences of growing up and growing outward into a world that wasn't built for us. We aren't separate from the participants and we're all learning how to be "good ancestors" during our time on earth in our physical bodies, at various stages of our journeys.

Lizzie states that with fierce love, "My belonging [in BGR] is not based on whatever I can do for XYZ, this capitalist transactional exchange of *I can make this contribution*." Our collective members and families have inherent worth and belonging, regardless of the role we each play or where we are in our growth. "We're all at different places," Gloria, another parent and BGR auntie, says, "but we recognize, one, that we're all growing and we welcome that, and we're not going to throw each other away because we're not perfect." There have been many moments when a collective member had to take a break from BGR, be it for one meeting or a year, and yet they still had a place in our group.

## PLAY AND JOY

Creative engagement has been part of BGR's pedagogy from the start. We made sure to have interactive programming that included games, art, discussions, and more. Yet in the beginning, we still fell prey to white supremacist tendencies to try to stuff as much *information* into our youths as possible. The urgency we felt to help our youths engage in activism and be educated about social justice made us want to push too much content in our workshops. In many anarchist and leftist circles that we have participated in, this focus on theoretical knowledge combined with protests, boycotts, and so on, is upheld as the gold standard for revolutionary work.

But we kept hearing from youths that the aspects of our programming they loved the most were when they were free to be creative and improvise, to be silly and playful. When we had swim days, learned group games, and got messy with art supplies, and especially when we took the kids on overnight campouts in the summer, youths showed as well as told us of their joy and excitement. We saw them put energy into each other and our work more deeply.

Listening to our youths, we realized that play and joy were not means to an end, not the sugar that helped the medicine of *real* learning go down. The play and joy *are* the goal. For Black and Brown girls and nonbinary youths, play and joy can be scarce resources. Hierarchical social systems strive to deny us these aspects of human life in order to keep us tired, destabilized, and subjugated. Our neighborhoods are deprived of parks, museums, and cultural centers. BIPOC youths, especially Black youths, are seen as older than they actually are, and therefore punished younger and not afforded a lengthy, playful childhood. And most BIPOC youths don't have the luxury of waiting until they are older to understand the harms that exist in the world. We experience them personally from a young age.

Black and Brown youths heal when they have the opportunity to play and have fun. Centering play in youth work and indeed all activism means that we are practicing *now* the world we wish to have in the future—a prefigurative politics. In *Undoing Border Imperialism*, Harsha Walia defines prefiguration as "the notion that our organizing reflects the society we wish to live in—that the methods we practice, institutions we create, and relationships we facilitate within our movements and communities align with our ideals."[2] We know that we wish to live in a world in which kids can be kids and develop at their own pace, and in which pleasure is equally available to everyone. As Grace asserts, "We also recognize that joy has always been crucially restorative for our peoples and an essential part of the resilience of our communities. Creating spaces of joy has literally always been how Black and Brown queer people have sustained ourselves throughout history and fluctuating degrees of violence or being targeted."

Around our third year, BGR began turning further toward this way of practicing youth work and intergenerational organizing. Today we rarely have traditional workshops with lots of talking at youths. Our programming mainly consists of joyful activities such as roller-skating, swimming, art making, and farming. We get into our bodies as much as possible and find ways to meet each other there, connecting through play. We believe play is a basic human need.

One illustration of how play became central took place during late spring 2020, at the height of the uprising following the murder of George Floyd by Minneapolis police. BGR organized a meetup for any families that wished to be in community together at a vigil in a park in North Portland. Hundreds of people were present, mostly adults, standing and sitting with signs, listening to a long line of speakers. It felt heavy.

The kids who were present had for months been learning

---

2. Harsha Walia, *Undoing Border Imperialism* (Oakland, CA: AK Press, 2013), 11.

remotely because of the pandemic, isolated from each other most of the time, yet they were constantly hearing news of our people being killed. It seemed to come naturally to them that when meeting up in person amid all the intensity, they wanted to play with each other. Rather than demanding that they and their families conform to the norms of typical protest behavior, several BGR organizers began to play with them. The organizers learned TikTok dances with the youths and formed a little crew of performers. They handed out bubble-making supplies and chalk, and the kids spent an hour writing and drawing beautiful messages all over the park against police violence and in support of Black lives. There was silliness *and* anger *and* conviction in these activities. As Lizzie, a parent and BGR organizer, put it, "You could see in the youths who were present, this sense of *I'm releasing something, and there are people around me who care about me and see me, and are mirroring back my joy at me.* Even in the midst of this really painful moment, they are feeling in their body."

In this example, play allowed us to connect with each other and gave the young people space to process what they were feeling. It offered them a chance to feel delight and participate in ways that were meaningful for *them*, not others. Simultaneously, play is one of the best ways we can engage in problem-solving. When we live in a society that includes terrible acts of inequity and brutality, it can be difficult to figure out paths to a better world. Imagination provides us with a platform to explore the unknown while in relationship with each other. We can try out different ways of being and discover what organically emerges that was unavailable to us via intellectual exercises.

❖ ❖ ❖

In his manifesto and guide to storytelling and imaginary play, *Grammar of Fantasy*, Italian communist, author, and children's educator Gianni Rodari sums up his views on the revolutionary nature of creativity in his chapter titled "Lenin's Grandfather." He recounts a story he heard about children in Russia who liked to sneak into their cousin Vladimir Lenin's grandfather's garden via a window versus the door.

> The wise Professor Blank (Lenin's grandfather on his mother's side) was very careful not to forbid this innocent fun and had firm benches placed beneath the windows so that the children could go in and out without the danger of breaking their necks. It seemed to me to be an exemplary way of placing oneself at the service of children's imagination.
>
> By using stories and those fantastic methods that produce them, we help children to enter reality through the window instead of through the door. It is more fun. Therefore it is more useful.
>
> Moreover, there is nothing to prevent anyone from having an impact on reality by means of more demanding For example: *What would happen if there were suddenly no more money to be found in the entire world, from the North Pole to the South?*"[3]

The state doesn't wish for us to be well enough to dream

---

3. Gianni Rodari, *The Grammar of Fantasy: An Introduction to the Art of Inventing Stories* (New York: Teachers and Writers Collaborative, 1996), 20.

of another way of living that excludes the state. We can see this in everything from the defunding of the arts and mental health programs, to the destruction of Indigenous healing and well-being traditions. We reclaim all sorts of ways to feel pleasure and envision a better future for ourselves.

Our leadership team strives to experience this playfulness and joy together as well, though again, it's not always easy. One of the main barriers to integrating these values in BGR is that everyone on our collective is already dealing with so much. Energy levels are low, and we can get stuck in feelings of crisis, scarcity, and burnout. We push back on these challenges by making food together, singing karaoke, celebrating birthdays, and processing and planning via theater of the oppressed and somatic exercises. Because our work is often hard, and because we continually experience violence and have to fight against the tide of white supremacist culture, emphasizing pleasure is a necessity. "I'm tired of my joy being resistance," Dani says.

> And I am tired of it being that for the youths too. So I'd rather see it as just a natural experience that everybody deserves. But also seeing the way that it serves people, and yes, serves us on a physiological level, on a mental level, and at the same time is a big relationship builder. If you can laugh with somebody, if you can kiki with somebody like you, if you can be weird with somebody, then it makes it so much easier to transition into the things that you don't always feel comfortable talking about with other people.

Sisterhood, fierce love, play, and joy are all deeply interrelated.

Kalie, a youth who came up through our programming and is now a member of the organizing collective, speaks to the impact of these values: "After the first [BGR] meeting, I just felt so amazing. I was finally home. I tend to bottle up a lot of my emotions around people. I don't let myself go, and I don't let myself have fun. But when I'm with BGR, I can just fully let myself be."

❖   ❖   ❖

Although this piece was written by claire barrera, it was a deeply collaborative and relational effort that included Ashnie Butler, Allie Dyer, Lizzie Fussell, Dani Mandley, Ash Martin, Grace McMickens, Gloria Pinzon, and Kalie Pinzon. Shoutout as well to other current and former BGR collective members: Noelle Al-Musaifry, Anayeli Diaz, Madeleine Harmon, Shantae Johnson, Akasha Lawrence Spence, Lara Pacheco, Iris Torres, and Lorraine Wilson. For more on BGR, see https://browngirlrise.org/.

claire barrera is an artist, educator, and activist based in Portland, Oregon. They coedit *When Language Runs Dry: A Zine for People with Chronic Pain and Their Allies*, and choreograph performance works, most recently the intergenerational piece *Grammar of the Imagination*. Currently they funnel their energy into antiviolence and youth liberation work, dance, and Dungeons and Dragons.

# COLECTIVA MUJERES SUBVERSIVAS: IN SOLIDARITY AND FRIENDSHIP

/

LORA GALORA

This story is like a bindweed, weaving together chronicles of urban oppression with legends of freedom, myths of music, and anecdotes of direct action. We revel in revolt, with love, reclaiming the wild garden within us all. We are Colectiva Mujeres Subversivas / Subversive Women's Collective. And you are too.

❀ ❀ ❀

There we were, in a squatted abandoned lot at a feral punk show in Querétaro City, deep in Carrillo, a neighborhood that was once full of flower farms, but has sadly been invaded by concrete factories. A place where the false flag of progress took precedence over the human lives that reside there. Yet humans are resilient. It's no surprise that this trampled community was the bastion of a thriving scene, back when punk was illegal. Back when distortion and dissonance were outlawed. The prohibition of wild music couldn't and wouldn't stick. No matter how many times you dig up dandelions, they always grow back. The community organized—and it keeps organizing. Freedom is a fight that never ends. Today those small deserted lots, full of broken bottles and broken promises, disguise fertile land ripe with the flowering seeds of friendship and rebellion that continue to swirl on the wind, carrying their dreams wherever they go.

"Mujeres Subversivas are born from one moment to the next in any space-time."[1] We give birth to each other, sprouting up

1. This line is excerpted from a poem by Gabriela Navajas Rojas titled *Brote Subversivo* (Subversive Outbreak), shared in full at the end of this piece.

from urban decay, from the rot of capitalistic malevolence, from the violence of toxic masculinity. We are the wild plants that grow up through the cracks of concrete, and one by one we guide each other back to the fertile lands of grassroots autonomy, mutual aid, horizontalism, and companionship. But even in the so-called anarchistic punk scene, our flowers get trampled in the form of microaggressions and petty competition. We find ourselves walking on eggshells around fragile egos. Our songs get talked over, our voices muted, until we have to scream just to be heard. Where the fuck is the solidarity?

That's how Mujeres Subversivas came into being, back in 2019. The first call, one of many, was initiated by Mara and Anita. Working with a cogendered collective, they organized a two-day event called Mujeres Subversivas: Anarcho-Feminist Action and Self-Defense. There was a DIY market, discussion about the zine "Accion y AutodefensAnarcofeminista" (Anarcho-Feminist Action and Self-Defense), self-defense class, documentaries, and workshops on interpersonal violence and teaching new forms of masculinity, screen printing, papermaking, and stencils, not to mention performances by lots of bands and a radical feminist theater troupe called Ollin Compani. Many people in attendance, though, got upset that the thespians took to the stage between bands and started disrespecting the powerful art being performed before them. The artists and actors were baring their souls and getting heckled for it. The rage in that moment sparked the fire for the femme-based collective Mujeres Subversivas. That same rage could still be felt under the rubble of the old flower fields.

Soy mujer y quiero ser poeta.

Quiero nombrar la violencia con flores en la boca.

Quiero ser de las que hacen que el mundo se acomode.

Quiero crear palabras que corten de tajo el otoño y de paso, la cabeza de algunos violadores.

Quiero decirles a mi madre,

a mis amigas y a todas ellas,

que estamos haciendo historia y es poesía porque son ellas,

Quiero ver que el fuego se propague por las fiscalías y no por las fábricas con ellas

Quiero que las balas apunten a Dios y no hacia ellas,

Quiero que reciten su llanto hasta que se haga lluvia,

quiero navegar junto a ellas,

quiero que el viento sople a favor de ellas,

quiero que los huracanes sean ellas,

quiero que la esperanza sea en ellas,

¡quiero que el mundo sea con ellas!

Y quiero, que nuestros corazones

se agiten de Amor,

de Rabia,

pero nunca de miedo …

Quiero que al menos estas palabras atraviesen el planeta y crezcan flores con espinas que muestren la fuerza de ser mujer, de ser poeta y de ser con ellAs.


I am a woman and want to be a poet.

I want to name violence with flowers in my mouth.

I want to be among those who bend the world to us.

I want to create words that cut off autumn, and along the way, the heads of some rapists.

I want to tell my mother,

My friends, and all of them,

That we are making history and because of them it is poetry.
I want to see fire spread through the prosecutors' offices and not
the factories where they [our mothers] work,
I want the bullets aimed at God and not at them,
I want them [our grandmothers] to utter their laments until they
become rain,
I want to sail with them,
I want the wind to blow in their favor,
I want them to be hurricanes,
I want them to be hope,
I want this world to be theirs!
And I want our hearts
To tremble with love,
With rage,
But never with fear …
At the least, I want these words to cross the planet and grow
thorned flowers that show the strength of being a woman, of being
a poet, of being them.[2]

❖ ❖ ❖

Gaby threw her words off the stage and into the hearts of the
crowd at this punk show, kindling their inner fires. The potent
rhythm of a drumbeat felt like the countdown to a blastoff.
It was followed by a screaming guitar riff and bass line that
resounded throughout the space. The music was throbbing,
sharp, raw, and direct. An all-femme mosh pit broke out,

---

2. *Reexistir* (Reexist) by Gabriela Navajas Rojas, a poem used in a song
by the band Filoso.

our bodies flying around in a blur of fishnets, patches, studs, glitter, chains, boots, eyeliner, and raised fists full of rings. Hugging each other passionately, we spun around to keep the chaotic energy moving. "Sharpen your knives! Sharpen your minds!" Gaby screamed into the mic, the voice of our fury, the voice of our solidarity. She ended with a body-shaking shriek. When the music ended and the musicians conferred about the next song, chatter bubbled up among us.

"Chingón [fucking awesome]!!!"

"Amigaaaa! What an epic day! First the Autonomy for Kids workshop and now this! Increíble!" Fist bump.

❈ ❈ ❈

Anita clapped her hands together. The game was starting in today's kids workshop. We lined the children up in a row, making the younger, rambunctious, and distracted Erizo the leader. He called the shots, directing the other kids to pass small foam mats—foamies, as we called them—along a path to get to the other side. No one else was allowed to speak. It took some coaxing on our behalf, reminding him now and again of the goal, and asking him what he should do next, but eventually he got all the other kids across.

We played again, but this time we changed the rules. Now everyone could share their ideas and work together collectively without a leader. Needless to say, the kids made it across much faster on the second pass. Then we all sat in a circle talking about the experience. How did it feel to have to listen to one single person in charge and not be able to voice your thoughts? What changed when no one was the leader and everyone could work together? Which version worked better? Gaby spoke about the difference between vertical and horizontal hierarchy. How working together collectively opened the space for new ideas and faster outcomes, not to mention that having your voice heard is important to everyone. Anita emphasized the importance of listening to others, and having the courage to speak up for yourself and those you care about, or those who aren't always able to speak up for themselves.

❋ ❋ ❋

We wrapped up the workshop and led the kids through the patio, past the parents sitting in the front room and into the kitchen of Casa de Vinculación Social (Social Connection House) to wash their hands. Casa de Vinculación is a social center in the heart of Carrillo. It's a large two-story house with ample front and back patios as well as a large garden.

Many collectives flow in and out of the space. Over time, a musical collective has taught guitar classes for kids, various exercise classes have been held, a psychologist offers care, and people built a sweat lodge out back. An environmental collective maintains the gardens. Several years ago, Casa de Vinculación organized and planted a community garden in an abandoned lot around the corner too. Recently, a couple of the collectives got together to form Micelio (Mycelium), which organizes around the issue of Querétaro's water, an especially poignant topic since 2022, when the state moved to officially privatize water rights. The state's plan has sparked many calls to action and a larger conversation about the future of water in Mexico.

The ship that is Casa de Vinculación is under the guidance of the formidable Mari Carmen, who provides a special space in a neighborhood that is frequently overlooked and overpowered by the industries that built over its flower fields and mesquite trees. Mujeres Subversivas started working with Casa de Vinculación in 2020. And now that the kids workshop had wrapped up, it was time to put everything away. But first snacks.

❖   ❖   ❖

The parents had prepared sliced fruit and tostadas with vegan toppings and salsas, and made sure that coffee and lemon verbena tea stayed hot on the stove. They sat in the next room around a big table chatting and opened up space for several of us to sit, while others began bringing the foamies back upstairs and putting away the art supplies. Mona, Ramona's mother, thanked us.

"This is such great work you all do. How did you get started?"

We looked around at each other.

"Well …" Mara started.

"Mara!" blurted out Fatx. "You're the connection for all of us."

Mara shrugged with a smile. "Well what can I say? I just wanted to be organizing with powerful feminists. And it all just came together."

Then Anita spoke up. "I remember the temazcal [sweat lodge] with Gaby and Pau that Yun organized with her collective, Casa Tonatzin Tlalli Temazcal." Yun gave her a wink. "Oh thank you, amiga, that felt like a metaphor for the birth of our collective. And then we all just came together from different parts of the city, from different backgrounds, different ages. Like the invitation was sent out, and everybody came running." Anita giggled with an excited hand gesture and elvish grin.

"And at just the right moment!" Leo jumped in, pointing at her. "One by one we gathered together, looked around, and realized we'd found something really special. Then later we found this space to work out of, Casa Vinculación, and everything just came together."

❖　❖　❖

Victoria, Erizo's mother, nodded with understanding. Lora came down from putting the foamies and art supplies away, finding the last empty seat at the table. There was curiosity in the eyes of Yun, whose boys Mateo and Geronimo were playing with the other kids out back. "OK, so explain to me more about your collective," Yun said with her warm smile. "Like what is it?"

The intention of Mujeres Subversivas, from the start, has been to create a network of women and femmes connected by common ideals, organized horizontally and in solidarity, to share feelings, thoughts, and the fire that rages within us all. To weave the world with our words, growing together up out of the concrete, sharing hardships and cultivating our wild ways within the world.

Fatx eagerly asserted, "I see our collective as a platform to know ourselves through each other. We come from all over the city as artists, teachers, painters, dancers, and poets, and together our actions create space to live out our ideals, dreams, rebellions, and passions. We all came to Mujeres Subversivas looking for change—in ourselves, in our community. We believe in building a better system, and we're doing the work to make it happen."

"One rebellious mural at a time!" blurted out Leo, laughing. "Mujeres Subversivas is based on friendship. We're about freedom and horizontal organizing. We're about solidarity and mutual aid. We teach each other lessons, from the kids to the adults and everyone in between. We're diverse and cross-generational. We even have a member from the other side of the border," Leo said, looking at Lora, who smiled, shrugged, and then gave her own answer in an accented Spanish.

"I see us as revolutionaries. We have strong personalities, we have conflicts, but at the end of the day, we all have the same goals. Freedom. Make the world a better place. And we each bring different ideas about how to accomplish those dreams. When we mix all of our ideas together, I like to think that we're able to bring something really special into the world."

❊ ❊ ❊

"Definitely," said Majo, the mother of José Carlos. "What other activities have you all put together?"

"The first event we put together as Mujeres Subversivas was with Polilla, who came up from Puebla to organize a big three-day event over the course of two weekends. The idea was a direct action on the street to create a feminist mural using stencils," Mara replied. "On the first day, we had a discussion about anarcho-feminist education. We shared ideas about strategies and working collectively. We spoke about bringing art and direct action into the public space.

"The next day, Polilla taught us how to use stencils. It was also a massive brainstorming day. We threw all of our ideas together. To start, we wanted to demonstrate freedom and autonomy, so we used a drawing of a bicycle to represent that. We wanted to be inclusive for all kinds of women, so we made the bike long with multiple seats to include a woman with a prosthetic leg. There was one person in high heels and another in boots to portray the spectrum of femininity. We also added a child to represent motherhood. The bicycle was shooting flames to represent the internal fire we all carry, and in the flames we'd written 'Existe Resiste' (Exist! Resist!).

"The next weekend, we got together for the third and final day to paint. We worked in groups to make the mural because the stencils were so large. That was in December 2020. Then in February, we got together and created another three murals."

"The murals were amazing," said Leo. "My grandparents even showed up! I was kinda scared about that at first, but it turned out great."

Gaby came in from washing the dishes. She wiped her hands on a tablecloth. "I really loved those events! It was a perfect balance of being organized yet spontaneous."

"Oh my goddess, yes," said Pau.

"Has anyone swept yet?" asked Fatx.

"Not yet," answered Gaby.

Leo got up and headed to the broom closet, leaving a space for Gaby to sit down.

One component of working with Casa de Vinculación was that we were responsible for cleaning the space after using it. There was no overt delegation of tasks for this. Instead, it always flowed organically. Putting away supplies, sweeping, mopping, dishes, and tidying. Usually another round of dishes. Making sure there was toilet paper in the bathroom, and finally, locking up afterward. This was part of working in collaboration with other collectives, forming a larger community of dreamers, organizers, artists, and healers.

"Yeah that event did have good flow," said Mara. "Then there was the lecture series we did on anarcho-feminism with writings from Peggy Kornegger.[3] We did one every month for four months. We got together and collaboratively created the flyer collages for each one."

"That was fun," said Lora. "It was hard too, because we all have such strong opinions, but I think we learned a lot about working together in those sessions."

"Then we stepped up our game with the Autonomía Para Niñxs [Autonomy for Kids] workshop," said Anita, "and twice a week!"

"Thank you again," said Mona. "It's been great for the kids to reconnect after all the craziness in the world."

We all kind of sighed and took sips from our coffee, or

---

3. Peggy Kornegger, "Anarchism: The Feminist Connection" (1975), Anarchist Library, https://theanarchistlibrary.org/library/peggy-kornegger-anarchism-the-feminist-connection.

grabbed another piece of fruit. The pandemic had been a bookmark in time for so many things, the collective included. During the quarantine, we organized an online self-defense class. Once we could meet up in person again, we started working with Casa de Vinculación. That was a whole new phase. We all had extra time, so we were meeting up almost every week, and sometimes more, to plan for the lecture series and organize for the M8 Women's March, which happens once a year in every major city across Mexico on March 8. We were part of a class on libertarian education and were dreaming up a workshop for children.

＊　＊　＊

"So what have you folks learned from all of your organizing?" Sebastian inquired

We grew pensive.

"Take notes!" said Gaby, which got a round of laughs and lightened the mood.

Then Lora spoke up. "I think we probably overorganized the lecture series. Turns out you can overdo it on the organizing end. We were meeting all the time, but we would get off topic and didn't get a lot done. Not always; sometimes our meetings were really productive, but at other times it was like four hours would just disappear without anything concrete happening."

"Yeah, there was a lot of self-induced stress," Fatx observed. "I think we've learned the importance of delegation and trust—to trust ourselves, trust each other. We don't all have to be there for a flyer collage, for instance."

Gaby built on that, saying that it was "finding a balance of organization and spontaneity. Honestly, I think a fast-approaching deadline can help everything come together. Everyone finds what needs to happen and gets it done."

"It's balance, like you said. You don't want an event so unorganized that no one knows what's happening and it's all chaotic," added Mara.

Leo put the broom away and popped back into the conversation. "I've learned that I wasn't the only one who wanted to do this. There are a lot of people who want to change things, who know there are better ways. We keep the faith and find what actions to take. And by doing that we connect with others who share that same internal desire to live better. I feel grateful that everything came together for all of us. That doesn't always happen for people who want it to."

"But that's what DIY is all about, right?" said Mara. "Do it yourself, start with a friend, find another, then another, and it all snowballs into the beautiful dream you have. And by organizing these small events, you never know who might come into the fold or who you're opening the door for."

"That's so true. I think we are making an impact, but we might not even see it. We might be blazing a path for someone for things they didn't even realize were possible. And we'll never know," Lora reflected. "Just like those who came before us will never know how important that first punk show was, or that first protest or first radical feminist theater performance. And it's never just one person. It's collective, it's community, it's the scene, it's everything. But regardless there's something inside of us that makes us do it."

Leo exclaimed, "Yes, that community weaving, where we

effect this small piece of the world, but it ripples out! From the individual to everyone's beautiful kids and the people who come to our events. We even make an impact on our friends and families with the actions we take."

"And it has an impact on ourselves as well," noted Pau. "Sharing, organizing together, it brings us out of ourselves and places us into the world. Like when you climb a mountain and you get a larger perspective of everything. We can start to see what we're doing. I think the closing party we threw for the anarcho-feminist lecture series brought that all together for me."

❧ ❧ ❧

That afternoon of the lecture series felt like a psychic hug from the collective. We were equals, smiling and happy. And we were fierce! We channeled our rage into stories sung as poems hurled into each other's hearts. We were vulnerable, opening up about our battles and crying over our wounds of war. We were furious, but we weren't alone. That made all the difference, and together we danced joy back into each other's lives, creating and sharing our art.

Mujeres Subversivas has been our call to action, solidified with the help of everyone there. Together we forge this liminal space, with open dialogue and an egalitarian spirit, carrying the torch for those who couldn't make it and those who first lit it to create a magical space where we feel protected, safe, and accompanied. Our work in collective has always been accomplished through horizontal organization and autogestión, which is a word that doesn't translate well.

DIY comes close. *Self-management* is what the dictionary says. Autogestión is a way to generate opportunity for yourself without a boss.

To open the party that marked the close of the lecture series we held a DIY market, where our friends bartered and sold their art—inspiring us with their energy and their fire. Once the space had filled with laughter, we gathered everyone together for the last lecture in our series, which included a slideshow, arts and crafts, and deep questions. We've always strived to bring a balance of tactical experience and theory to our events, and this one was no different.

We concluded with the open mic, which without over-organizing, was spontaneous and organic. At first, we were anxious there wouldn't be enough time or that nobody would want to perform (despite the fact that the open mic was listed on our flyer). As it turned out, between ourselves and those who had participated in the lecture series there was no shortage of performances: poems and theoretical musings were read out of scribbled handmade notebooks, instruments were played, and voices offered the songs they'd been waiting to share, some melodic and some dissonant.

The first act to light up the mic was Power Animala, an all-femme rap group that inspired our bodies into motion with dynamic beats. Powerful verses made our hearts run wild. Then Fer shared a poem addressed to the trash human who'd wasted her time while she'd let her own talents languish. Josi filled the microphone with a poignant story about a person who tried to cut off their colorful wings and wanted to control their magical dreams. Roux gave a solo rap performance about the time she was metaphorically drowned by a relationship that kept her glow from lighting up the sky. Leo took our breath away with her exposed, passionate body. As she danced and twerked, we saw parts of ourselves that we've denied, and the desire to rebel. Musa bewitched us with her lyrics full of rage, love, and rebellion on ukulele rhythms that transported us to mysterious dimensions. Fatx closed by creating the space for us to pause and reflect, to search for ways to process emotions, with an interactive zine full of love.

"That open mic was like looking into an open heart. It felt like standing before the mirror of all my sisters as we rewrite our history as womyn," Pau asserted.

The beauty of her words stunned us into silence. We looked into our empty drinks. Then Anita slapped her hands on the table, "Well, I'm going to go mop!"

And we all laughed.

"Does anyone still have unwashed dishes? I'll do round two."

"Thank yous" were handed out along with the dirty cups and small plates. Yun looked around the table at us and then asked, "So what comes next for all of you?"

"We're a work in progress, a movement, constructing reality through the people we meet. We are a circle of trust. We want to change, to try new things. We learned from the lecture series that too much organizing can get in the way," Leo answered. "But we're still here. We still want to put events together; we just want them to flow more organically."

Gaby explained that "the difficulties and dramas that we faced in the past were part of the process, and they've made all of our friendships so much stronger. I've seen us change both individually and as a group."

"Truly. With each cycle we go through, we get deeper, find more space," affirmed Fatx. "Now what's next? Where do we go from here?"

Just then Pau entered the room with the mop. "Amigas! I think where we go from here is to the show!" She turned to the parents in the room. "Are y'all coming too? It's at the city museum downtown. It's a great venue to bring the kids to."

"Yeah, we're definitely coming," said Yun.

"Us too!" chimed in Victoria and Sebastian at once.

"Great, let's go!"

❖   ❖   ❖

We finished up the last of the chores, gathered up the children, and piled into various vehicles to caravan together downtown. The city museum was a collision of the past and present. Its stone Spanish architecture of the colonized past met with modern mood lighting of the present while powerful artwork hung in stark contrast on white plaster walls. It was an unlikely venue, usually reserved for fine art exhibitions and gatherings of Querétaro's well-to-do. The building had an outdoor patio built into the interior, and that's where the show was taking place. So while the Spaniards had forced their culture onto the diverse Indigenous peoples of what is now Mexico, we were spreading our own culture in this place that now belonged to the upper class, the oppressor class. It was a strange dichotomy indeed, but we were here to break the space and claim it as our own—at least for a night anyway.

Gaby took to the stage, grabbing the mic and channeling

our fury and rage, our solidarity and friendship.

❋   ❋   ❋

Las mujeres subversivas nacemos de un momento a otro y en
cualquier espacio-tiempo.
Emergemos en el instante que nos re/conocemos
niñas
madres
abuelas
hermanas
tías
amigas
educadoras
humanas
En ese momento,
en el que nos asumimos mujeres aún sabiendo
que estamos ante un sistema que nos dice
las otras,
las olvidadas,
las anuladas.
Es ese momento,
en el cual nos cuestionamos acerca de todo aquello que no nos
permite ser
y que ahora sabemos,
lograremos arrancarlo de nosotras de la misma manera que
podemos
y deseamos hacerlo de este mundo.
Es ese momento,
en el que descubrimos nuestra capacidad

de acción, de transformación y de Resistencia,
Es ese momento,
en el que se nace mujer subversiva.
Nosotras, las Mujeres Subversivas, somos aquellas que pueden
mirarse a sí mismas desde las demás personas,
aquellas que nos hemos organizado y autoeducado en colectivo,
desde una educación que nos libera y nos permite ir construyendo
nuevas rutas encaminadas a nuevos destinos;
a nuevas realidades,
a nuevos vínculos,
a nuevas sociedades,
sin Dios,
sin jerarquías,
sin patrones,
sin competencia,
sin división.
Con (A)mor y Rebeldía
¡Qué vivan las mujeres subversivas!

Mujeres Subversivas are born from one moment to the next in any
space-time.
We emerge the instant we recognize ourselves.
girls
mothers
grandmothers
sisters
aunts
friends
educators
humans
In that moment,
when we embrace ourselves as women despite knowing that we

face a system that calls us
the other,
the forgotten,
the voided.
It is that moment,
in which we question ourselves about all that does not allow
us to be
and that we now know,
we will be able to uproot from ourselves the same way we will
and want to uproot it from this world.
It is that moment,
in which we discover our capacity
for action, transformation, and resistance.
It is that moment,
in which the subversive woman is born.
Mujeres Subversivas are those who can see ourselves as others do,
Those who have collectively organized and self-educated ourselves,
with an education that liberates and allows us to build new paths
to new destinations,
to new realities,
to new connections,
to new societies,
without God,
without hierarchies,
without bosses,
without competition,
without division.
With love and rebellion
¡Long live Mujeres Subversivas!

* * *

Mujeres Subversivas was founded in 2019 and is based in Querétaro, Mexico. There are currently seven members, though they are looking forward to expanding. They can be reached on Facebook at Mujeres Subversivas Acción y Autodefensa Anarcofeminista. Amor y rabia hermanxs!

# PINK PEACOCK: LAVISHLY ACCESSIBLE

/

## MOISHE HOLLEB
## IN CONVERSATION WITH
## ALICE ROSS

The Pink Peacock | עוואַפֿ עוועזאַר יד began as a mutual aid project in 2020. On Rosh Hashanah 5782 | September 2021, after months of hard manual work, the collective opened a queer, Yiddish, anarchist feminist, anticapitalist café and infoshop on Victoria Road in Glasgow. The space was run entirely by volunteers, and everything—from food to events to the online shop—was always pay-what-you-can down to £0. In late Sivan 5783 | June 2023, amid astronomical price increases for rent and utilities, and with collective members all suffering from the latest stage of capitalistic collapse and nationalistic self-destruction across the United Kingdom, the Pink Peacock closed its doors. The following conversation with cofounder Moishe (Misha) Holleb | השם (עשימ) בעלאָה (he/him/ער/מיא) took place a few months earlier.

I first met Misha, and the Pink Peacock's other cofounder, Joe Isaac (she/her), during Rosh Hashanah 5780 | September 2019.[1] The Jewish New Year falls at the end of summer, traditionally the period when we've harvested our crops, and all the seeds we sowed during the year have come to fruition (or not). We pause there, on a threshold, before entering the transition into the dark, dormant part of the cycle. For me it's a time to reflect on our actions and choices, and think about what's important, what needs to change, and what we want to do and be in the coming year. Misha and Joe didn't know me. We'd connected virtually through one of those loose, fragile networks of anarchist-adjacent thinkers that exist in many places. They shared a wonderful celebratory meal with me that night in their home, making me feel relaxed and welcome

---

1. While Joe isn't interviewed here, I want to honor her wonderful work and contributions throughout the project.

in a completely new (to me) kind of Jewish community. On my way home to another city about two hours away, waiting in Glasgow's brutalist central bus station at midnight, I felt tender and openhearted, quietly in awe.

That first time we met, I will always remember Misha saying that he wanted to start a Jewish anarchist café. It sounded lovely, but I couldn't imagine how such a thing could really happen. I thought it was a statement that told me something sweet about my new friend, not about the world we live in, gray, skeptical, and hard. As it turned out, it was both.

The Pink Peacock project began about half a year later, during the first COVID-19 lockdown in 2020, when everything changed. Misha and Joe started by running regular deliveries of homemade vegan Jewish food from their home to others, then an online art and infoshop, and beautiful, inclusive, online ritual events, including a weekly group discussion and blessings for Havdalah (the closing of Shabbat and onset of a new week). I took part in some of these, in various moods—often sad, sometimes hopeful, perpetually grateful—and felt the significance of the ritual in a way I hadn't appreciated before: creating a sacred time-space together, grounding ourselves through our senses. In that desperately frightening, isolating time, it was wonderful to share those moments (and conversations about ghosts and love, plants and *Star Trek*, and much more) with far-flung people through the hub of the Peacock. I've drawn inspiration and learned so much from the various Pink Peacock events I've attended since then. Being around the Peacock taught me about food, justice, gender, magic, and Yiddish as well as new ways of thinking about work and social relations, this world, and the world to come.

During that time, I met people from all across the globe who asked me if I knew about the Peacock. They'd tell me enthusiastically that they'd been there once, or been at virtual events, or planned to make the trip there one day. Then, invariably, they'd share their astonishment that such a place could exist: Really, a luxuriously queer, fabulously accessible, Yiddish anarchist space where you could eat delicious bagels with carrot lox for free? It sounded, we all agreed, like a dream.

I thought a lot about those conversations when the Peacock's closing was announced—in the grieving days, feeling numb, discouraged, and lost, connecting with strangers again, this time through the lyrical tributes that we poured into the unfeeling void of social media and gentler circles of group chats. It felt miraculous when the space opened; it now feels impossible that it's gone. New parts of me, parts that I cherished, had grown up wrapped around its structure like vines.

"Like a dream" echoed in my head, reminding me of the closing passage of socialist poet William Morris's classic novel *News from Nowhere* (1890), in which the narrator experiences a postrevolutionary, utopian society full of happy, fulfilled people who have long ago dispensed with money and authority, sharing freely while taking pleasure in creative, domestic, and agricultural pursuits. The story ends abruptly when our protagonist wakes up at home and realizes they've been asleep the whole time: "[I'm] trying to consider if I was overwhelmed with despair at finding I had been dreaming a dream; and strange to say, I found that I was not so despairing. Or indeed *was* it a dream?" They think about the last look one of their new friends gave them and how it seemed to say,

> Go back again, then, and while you live you will see all
> round you people engaged in making others live lives
> which are not their own, while they themselves care
> nothing for their own real lives—men who hate life
> though they fear death. Go back and be the happier
> for having seen us, for having added a little hope to
> your struggle. Go on living while you may, striving,
> with whatsoever pain and labour needs must be, to
> build up little by little the new day of fellowship, and
> rest, and happiness. ... Yes, surely! and if others can
> see it as I have seen it, then it may be called a vision
> rather than a dream.

This is how I feel today: "not so despairing," at least most
of the time. I'm writing this less than a month after the
café closed its doors for the last time, and days before the
first mutual aid free meal share that I'm now organizing in
my area. Rosh Hashanah is still a couple of months away,
but again I have the feeling of standing on a threshold. I am
remembering and honoring the Pink Peacock, and as I do so,
I try to look ahead to our possible futures and back to the past
we shared. I know that others saw it, lived it, and felt the way
I felt; it was a vision and not a dream.

*There's so much that's important and unique about the café! Yet I know from being a regular visitor that both your accessibility policies and COVID safety processes are especially thorough, really considered, and an essential part of the way that the space operates.[2] Accessibility seems to be a key, guiding principle. So I was wondering about your influences. Were there are any texts, places, or experiences that were inspiring for you, or informed any aspects of the policies you've put in place around accessibility—or negative examples that demonstrated the need to do things differently?*

It was obvious to us from the beginning that accessibility would be a priority. We follow the social model of disability and accessibility: everyone has access needs, and they all deserve to be lavishly met.

Money is an access issue, and that's always been one of the fundamental principles of the café: that it's free. That came from our experiences of food insecurity. I remember the first time I was given free food in a similar way; it was summer 2011, I was about twenty-one, and my band was doing a DIY tour circuit with a bunch of anarchist punks. We were hungry, and someone said there was free food at a church every Wednesday or whatever; they gave away food, no questions asked, with no means testing. So we went and got fed there—and that changed my whole life. I realized that this was what I needed to be doing too. Soon I got involved with Food Not Bombs in East London, and that was even better than the church because it wasn't Jesus-y. The church people were nice—they weren't preaching or proselytizing—

---

2. For the full list and detailed descriptions of Pink Peacock's accessibility policies, see https://pinkpeacock.gay/accessibility/.

but churches can be alienating just because they're churches. But just seeing it happen, this practice, showed me that it was possible and essential. It's a basic human thing that people need to eat, and yet it costs money, so some people can't. And it's really important for the café to meet that need, especially because so often, both for Jewish and queer spaces, money is a barrier to entry and accessing community as well as food.

On other accessibility needs, there are so many different sides to it. Of course there are all the physical and sensory needs, which is what people often think of first. And then there are mental and social access needs. Things like you don't have to read Hebrew to come to our Seder. You don't have to look a certain way, or be between eighteen and thirty-four, to be treated with dignity as a queer person. You don't have to know all about gender theory and what your own gender stuff is in order to come talk to us about trans stuff. We didn't do a lot of reading theory. At the start, it was just Joe and I, and neither of us were up on crip theory; it was just, we know that these are barriers and so we're going to look at how we can reduce them. This wasn't a point of principle—the not reading. It would've been good if we had read more and known more; it just happens that we didn't do a lot of reading first. We didn't have time.

Our main influence has been constant feedback, both from our volunteers and other people in the community. Some things, I think, we did a really good job on, and other things, we did a bad job, and people told us and we learned from it. Joe and I are both autistic, and I've got other mental health stuff, which gave us some awareness of how equipped spaces are or aren't to deal with anything that's not normative. So mostly it was just empathy. We had the desire to be in and provide an accessible space, and the knowledge that disabled people are disproportionately likely to be poor and hungry, and that queers are disproportionately likely to be disabled, and so on. It was just knowing that people need a thing and so we try to make the thing happen.

*Could we talk a bit about communication between the collective members and other volunteers, and how people take responsibility and ownership around improving things in terms of accessibility? Are there any examples of someone sharing a new idea or suggestion on meeting an access need, and how has that gone?*

One of the first things that I say to new volunteers is that their dignity, comfort, and safety are what's most important. So if they're volunteering and there's something they don't want to do, they shouldn't be doing it; we can get somebody else to do it. Some people love to do dishes, some people love counting out coins, and some people are happy to clean the toilet because they love cleaning. The collective works.

It usually takes collective members some time before they really take ownership of the project because it's just so unusual that we're like, "OK, we've welcomed you in and now this space is yours as much as it's mine." It takes people a little while to really believe that. But then once they do, they start to make changes and make things better.

So, for example, people are constantly organizing and reorganizing the storage areas in the back to make things accessible. That might not be the most obvious accessibility thing for everyone, but it is for us, because now it's so much easier to find what you're looking for and it's not stressful anymore. One of the collective members made allergen charts. Somebody installed a bunch of shelving, and then we told him the shelves were too high—he's tall, and a lot of us are small—and he was like, OK!, and adjusted them straightaway so that it's easy for us all to reach stuff. And then we have one really tall person in the collective, and when they first joined, they found that some of the door frames were too low for them, so they asked, "Can we get some big bright yellow stickers or tape that's really visible so that I don't hit my head?" Obviously that was such an easy thing to accommodate, but as a short king, I just didn't think of it until it came up.

There are a lot of examples around neurodivergence too. We decided early to have autism-friendly days—low-sensory days where we wouldn't play music—but we changed from playing white noise to playing other things that are less harsh like birdsong because of the collective's feedback.

There are always potentially conflicting access needs as well, and I think that for the most part, we navigate those pretty well considering that we have no resources and we're all tired volunteers. For instance, the dog-free day: we have one dog-free day a week, and it works really well for most people who don't want to be around dogs. But it doesn't work for people who are extremely allergic to dogs because there are dogs in the space the rest of the time, and because we're clear that service dogs are welcome all the time, even on dog-free days. So if you're extremely allergic to dogs, then that is an access issue that at the moment, there's nothing we can really do about it because we've decided that we're going to prioritize the need of someone who has a service dog. And it sucks that we can't do both, but we can't do both.

So there are problems that we haven't solved yet. When we first started out, Joe and I expected it would be hard work to make the space accessible. Because basically nowhere else does it so thoroughly, we thought that it must be really difficult and expensive. And it's not. So much of it is so easy. Like, the lighting in the cafe is great, it works for the broadest umbrella group of people: it's bright enough that you can read at night when there's no natural light, but not so bright that it gives anyone who has sensory issues headaches or anything like that.

*I like the privacy curtains as well—you have these cute lacy-black curtains over the lower part of the windows so that plenty of light comes in, but you don't feel like you're sitting in a display window on the street, and they're not blackout curtains so it doesn't feel weird. It feels cozy and safer as a queer space.*

Thank you! Both of those things, the lights and curtains, really required little thought and not a lot of money to make them work, and you install them and then they're there forever. And there are so many access things that are like that. Such as installing a ramp—wheelchairs are always the first thing people think about, so installing a ramp is the kind of thing that's in the general public's mind. You install the ramp once and it's done. It's there for years and years before you need to replace it. So it's kind of pathetic that there isn't step-free access everywhere. I mean, it's different if all you have is a space that's up or down a flight of stairs in one of these old historic buildings where it's almost impossible if you don't have heaps of money and space to install an elevator. But for anywhere that's on the ground floor, if it doesn't have step-free access, that's really lazy and embarrassing, and there are so many places where they just haven't bothered. We installed our main ramp for the cost of concrete.

*Interestingly, I think some of the policies that are in place primarily because of accessibility also make such a big difference in terms of making the café space so special; they incidentally make it stick out against the mainstream experience of going to cafés in the capitalist hellscape. Like the lighting, and also the efforts you make to reduce noise by having soft furnishings, tablecloths, and so on. From my viewpoint, I come into the Pink Peacock and just notice how much more pleasant it is to be there. When I go to other places that are supposed to be nice and luxurious, often everything in there consists of hard, uncomfortable surfaces that reverberate noise. And as somebody who, as far as I know, doesn't have any specific sensory issues or particular communication difficulties, it's still just unpleasant and makes me feel angry because I know that, for instance, my deaf friend can't be in those environments, and there are so many other people who would struggle or have a horrible time in spaces like that.*

Even people who have no reason to be angry about it—people who don't have that empathy or understanding, and don't have any sensory issues—find those environments stressful. They're meant to be stressful. It's meant to keep table turnover high—that's why those cafés are built like that, especially the big corporate ones. By design, they don't want you lingering. And so this is something that we always knew we needed to do: make the café as comforting and welcoming as we can, and make sure people know that you don't need to spend any money to be here or stay as long as you like.

*The café has come about in a time and place where it's much needed. It's been sorely needed both in terms of the growing poverty in this part of the world, and the many kinds of insecurity and inequality that have been brought to light during COVID, and neither of those things look like they're going away. While the lockdowns are over, the cost of everything is rising, and so is food insecurity, so if anything, it's getting worse and worse right now in the United Kingdom.*

Especially at the beginning, we had a lot of people who had obviously never taken a COVID test; they didn't have access to them because they're street homeless, or because there were language barriers that meant that they don't interact with pharmacies or the Scottish government website. So I've shown dozens of people how to take their first COVID test— which was upsetting because I'm not a medical professional and I'm not really qualified to do this—and then sometimes those people would have a positive result, and then I'm the one who's giving them medical advice, saying here's what you need to do so that you can recover and not transmit it to anybody else. We get told all the time at the Pink Peacock that we're the only place asking people to take tests; people look at us like we're insane when we ask them to take COVID tests, even when they were easily available for free.

It seemed like, generally speaking, both anarchist and mainstream venues were thinking more about accessibility during the period where we were coming out of lockdowns.

But soon, a lot of people just wanted to forget about COVID. There was a really welcome pivot to making stuff available online, and I'm sad that it hasn't persisted for the most part, even among leftists. I'm so upset that queer spaces in this country failed so badly at any kind of pandemic protocol. I have expectations of leftist and queer spaces that maybe I don't have for Jewish community spaces here, just because the Jewish community is so small in Glasgow. But in leftist and queer circles, I've seen people—at least those in charge of spaces and organizing events—very, very quickly abandon pandemic measures. I mean, like, summer 2020, abandon them and never look back. I don't really go to queer things anymore because so many queer spaces and events don't have even the smallest nod to COVID hygiene.

As a community, haven't we learned anything from the AIDS crisis? The parallels are so obvious in terms of the things that you can do. Being airborne, COVID is even more contagious and easier to transmit, but what you can do is use protection—masks, air purifiers and ventilation, and nasal sprays—and get tested regularly. And especially if you're in riskier situations, get tested. And the fact that this parallel is not being drawn on in any kind of mainstream way is disturbing to me. I feel like we've forgotten our recent history, and at the expense of people's lives. People die because it's uncomfortable to remember.

*I would say that people seem to have forgotten not only the 1980s and 1990s but things that were so much in our general public awareness just two and three years ago as well: COVID prevention, and the widespread concern around things like food insecurity and insecurity of places for people to live. Certainly where I live, at the start of the lockdown there was this huge wave of general awareness that many people in our community were struggling, people who couldn't work and couldn't get furlough, people who couldn't risk going out to shops, and people who had suddenly found themselves trapped in unsafe situations. And it felt like everybody was worried about that. People were pulling together and getting together informal food delivery services; there was one that I helped with for a while, getting meals to people who were experiencing food insecurity. But many of those things have gradually disappeared, and now so much of the city feels like it's business as usual, and surely those problems haven't just gone away. Do you think it's that fatigue sets in?*

Yeah, there's fatigue, and there's exhaustion, because we've been going through and are still going through a pandemic and a lot of grief, and I think our collective capacity to deal with all of this is really weak right now. There's this sense of fatalism: What can we do?

*And yet in that extremely hard time, you've created this space!*

I'm not doing any other activism. This is all I'm doing, and that way, it will be sustainable and I can be reliable, rather than trying and failing to show up for everything that I care about. I make sure, as best I can, that there's food for people to eat and the café is open as much as possible, and I don't do anything else.

*What are some of the things that make it possible to keep it open, to sustain it and the collective? The decisions you've mentioned, thinking about sustainability and commitment, make me feel like this is a question that relates to accessibility too.*

Support. It's been so important, right from the start, that we had a lot of support both from people here in the Southside and a wider community online. We would be nothing without that. At the beginning of the pandemic, when we didn't have any space and we weren't sure whether this was going to work, we posted online that we were going to try doing food deliveries for people in our postal code for pay-what-you-want down to nothing. There were two separate links: here's where you place an order, and here's where you can send us money if you want to, but you don't have to, and we won't know if you do or not because we're not checking. We will just bring you food, and if you don't pay for it that's fine. And we did a few delivery days throughout spring 2020, and every time we made enough money to pay for our material costs—not our labor, but our material costs—except for the last time. So we posted about that on social media, just saying, "Hey, we didn't quite make up the costs this time, but we served eighty meals," or whatever it was, "and if you can help us cover the costs, here's the link," and people immediately did. We don't always get that kind of response now. But that really is what made things possible in the beginning.

We have the best customers and supporters. The customers who come to the café are overwhelmingly lovely. And online as well—there is a lot of bad-faith interaction on social media, and there are people out there who hate us and persistently harass us, and that is really depressing and actively makes me less able to engage. But the other side of it is people saying about the project, and our accessibility and COVID safety stuff, "I'm not in Glasgow, but I love and support you, and I wish somebody was doing this in my city." We hear that all the time.

*People who haven't even tasted the carrot lox—which is delicious, by the way—love you! This also relates to something I wanted to ask you about: social relations and what the café project has to offer, particularly from an accessibility viewpoint, in terms of changing, reshaping, or opening up those relations. You show people what's possible in the context of food and drink and accessible spaces, but are there ways that you're showing what's possible interpersonally?*

A lot of the volunteers at the café are disabled, and it's really important to us that we are supportive—not just "tolerant" or "accepting," but genuinely supportive of each other. So if someone's having a pain day and can't come in that day, or if they're here but they need to go home early, or they don't want to go home but they need to sit down for the rest of their shift instead of being on their feet, we say, "OK, great, do that." And that's been such a learning curve for all of us, to be in an environment where you can actually state your needs and have them met. That just doesn't happen most places. So that's one social thing that we're trying to shift for all the collective members—the way we think about labor and rest, and prioritizing the well-being of the workers above everything else. It always feels bad to close the café on a day when we're supposed to be open, but we are always so clear that we will close the café rather than have somebody working there who's not well in whatever way. So if you're working and you need to stop, and there's nobody else who can do it, then we'll close, and that's better than you being here and having a bad time.

It's also hard that nobody is telling each other when to take a break because we're all in charge of our own needs and boundaries. We're always trying to encourage each other to identify and state those boundaries, to say, "Hey, I need to sit down" or "I need to go home" or "I can't commit to this today," and we're getting better at it. And hopefully we do notice things with each other, like if I'm getting tired today or burning out generally, somebody will notice that and say something, but not necessarily so. There's no one who's going to "manage you" in that way because there are no managers.

*Right, I think it's important to note, though, that having those things—hierarchy and managers—which exist in "regular" jobs, doesn't necessarily mean that a worker is safer that way, or that their well-being is any better or being looked out for; it can be quite the opposite. Because the praxis that you're describing, genuinely putting the volunteer workers' health and well-being first, is incredibly far from the norm in paid work contexts. Even in public-facing jobs, you'll regularly see people at work who are visibly physically unwell and absolutely should not be at work doing those tasks right now, and it's so bad for everyone.*

Right, and that's just the visible things! There's always pain and exhaustion and mental health stuff that you can't necessarily see as well, and whether or not it's a public health concern, those people are absolutely not being looked out for and told that it's OK to stop, or take a long break, or go home.

We try to have a good collective culture around this, and I actually think we were better at it before but now we've slipped into being shit about taking breaks. Some people can be—definitely myself included—reluctant to take breaks, and actually stop and rest when they do take them. It's hard, and we're working on it, and we all know that we should be better at it, but we're also constantly understaffed. It would be easier to take breaks if we had enough people to cover everything, but we don't. So we're always pushing ourselves because we care, you know—it's important to us to stay open and keep making the food.

For me, one way that I navigate the mental gymnastics around taking care of myself and valuing my rest—because I want to be at that place—is reminding myself that if I burn out, then I can't help, and in fact then I'll be a burden on the collective because I need support too and that's not good for anybody. The idea of being a "burden" for needing support is fucked, but if leveraging my own internalized ableism works, then it works. And another tactic that I have is modeling: reminding myself that I'm trying to model the behavior that I want to see, so I'm a role model to you and you're a role model to me, and we constantly reproduce and strengthen our own social norms here in our milieu. So that means that it's my responsibility—not only to myself, but to everyone else—to model good behavior and our values, which includes resting when I'm sick or tired. Taking my breaks reminds other people to take theirs as well as giving me the rest that I need.

Another thing on social relations, and something I'm really proud of that the café does, is we shift the paradigm away from capitalist assumptions. People come in and order food, and we tell them the suggested total—people are regularly baffled by that as an idea. Sometimes they're like, "How do I pay it forward?" And we say, "You give us some money, and it goes into making the things." And they say, "No, I want to buy the next person a coffee," and we have to tell them that's not how this works. It's a small but really important distinction. The pay-it-forward system would be, say, you pay it forward for a coffee, I put a coffee token in the coffee jar, and then someone can get a free coffee with this coffee token. So first of all, that means that there is only free coffee if someone has paid and the token is in the jar. So that immediately doesn't fit with what we do because we will give you free coffee no matter what. If nobody pays, we will just give away free coffee until we run out of money and then that's it. And we accepted that in the beginning.

But second of all, the pay-it-forward model is built around the pay-it-forwarder feeling good, more than it is about the person receiving it and being able to do so with dignity. Obviously, having a pay-it-forward system is better than nothing—it's better than people not being able to access your thing at all, which is the case with most places, so I don't want to shit on people who do use it because they are trying to do a good thing. But think about how it is for the person receiving that. Like, do they have to take the token, or point to the thing and be asked to pay, and then say, "No, sorry, can I have it for free?" It draws attention to their poverty, which breeds shame and self-exclusion.

So we say, we will give you food no matter what. Here is how you can pay if you would like to, and you don't have to, and as best as we can, we're not going to watch you make that decision—that's why we keep the donation box away from the counter. You receiving the food or coffee has nothing to do with how much you can or can't pay. So we're shifting that socially for so many people. Sometimes people don't know how to receive free food because there's so much shame and stigma about receiving "charity." Making it accessible has to mean making it as dignified and easy as possible because you've got to remove these barriers of shame.

There's also something that we can see happening with those people who can and do pay. You can see something kind of flicker in their eyes. You say, "The suggested total is £6, but you can pay what you want down to zero," and they go, "Oh, OK, I'll just pay the £6." They're clearly not used to hearing that payment is optional, and I think this shows people that it is possible. It's possible to have this space—a space that does need money to function, but where the prices aren't set based on what we're selling; they're based on what you can afford. That feels like a social thing that we're changing.

We haven't really talked about feminism explicitly, but we have been talking around it. I think there's a lot to be said about caring and nurturing work, and what kinds of labor are more likely to be undervalued, and about food and all the different kinds of work that go into food, and what gets celebrated or not. There's that old but really good poster that says something like "Everybody wants to do the revolution, nobody wants to do the dishes." All kinds of organizing are important, but you can't have the revolution if there's no food. The work that we're doing at the café is capacity-building work: when we feed somebody, it means that they can do something else with their time. Because when you're hungry, you can't do anything else, you're just surviving. We can give people capacity. And maybe what they choose to do with that extra capacity is something awful! But I know that most of the time, it isn't—and even if it was, everybody deserves food.

That's also why the anarchist angle is something we're always up front about; we foreground the fact that this is an anarchist project, this is one avenue of anarchist organizing. And that means there'll always be someone who asks us, "Oh, but doesn't anarchism mean rioting and violence and chaos and disorder?" That's such a teachable moment. It's an annoying question, but we've been asked it so many times that we've got good answers now.

*That means education is another thing that you're providing for people. This kind of nonjudgmental education in political spaces is in short supply, and I think, also good feminist and accessibility praxis.*

I hadn't really thought about the space being educational outside the literature we stock, but yeah. So much of the education is social, like explaining anarchism, explaining Jewish stuff, health stuff. I talk to a lot of older gays about trans issues. It's just answering questions.

*From my point of view, another aspect of anarcha-feminist praxis, which is also accessibility praxis, is that you've committed to being a dry and all-ages-friendly place. I used to work in an extremely male-dominated workplace in tech a few years back before the pandemic, and all the social events centered around drinking. And it felt like it was always me and one or two other female workers who had to say,*

*"Hey, have you ever thought that maybe this isn't equally accessible to everyone? Do you know that there could be reasons why some people might not want to—or might not be able to—go get drunk with their male boss and their 90 percent male workforce and be in a situation where they're all drunk?" That really seemed like it was so new to people—the idea that alcohol isn't great for equality and accessibility.*

Exactly, yeah, and queer spaces here generally have the same problem of things revolving around alcohol and nightlife, which means there's nowhere to go if you don't want to drink.

*Right, so the café is a place you can come to if you're queer and in recovery, you're too young to go to a bar, pregnant or trying to get pregnant, don't drink for religious reasons, have caring responsibilities, or don't want to be around drunk people because of trauma. And there are also all kinds of issues around communication: for anyone who has any kind of difficulty with speech or hearing, or is using a language that isn't their first language, in places with loud music and drinking, it can be really difficult to interact. That can be a real invisible social barrier, and it's so important that you're providing an alternative.*

*I feel really inspired by our conversation; it's given me a lot to think about and new ways of considering accessibility as a concept. So thank you! To wrap up, do you have a piece of advice to share. Is there one thing you wish you'd known three years ago, or one thing you'd tell other organizers not to forget?*

I think the things I wish I'd known at the start and things I think other people need to know are maybe different. What I wish someone had told me is really specific and kind of depressing. I wish I'd been prepared for the amount of vitriol and harassment that we get from so-called leftists. We were prepared for antisemitism from Nazis, and queerphobic shit and TERFs, and cop harassment, and being slagged off in the *Sun* [a reactionary tabloid newspaper], and that kind of thing—which all happened. And we were also quasi-prepared for parasocial stuff from lonely people. But I was not prepared for being doxxed by people who called themselves antifascist. I was not prepared for the unhinged rumors about us, or people sharing my address online, or stalking my mother's Facebook in the name of trying to prove how rich my Jewish family supposedly is. So those are possibilities—realities—far more than I thought they were. And that's really sad. But knowing that ahead of time would have been helpful.

My perception of what people need to hear, though, is easier. You're probably worried that you don't know what you're doing, and that's OK. Do it anyway and you'll figure it out. It's so much better to do it and fumble and have things be a bit slower than you want than to not do it at all because you feel like you're not an expert or it won't be perfect immediately.

But also, I don't want to be unrealistic about this; there are reasons that we were able to succeed. First, having enough people in the collective. There was a point at the start when it was only the two of us, me and Joe, and we have different abilities so that meant there were specific things that only one person could do, and it was immediately obvious that even with neither of us having another job or childcare responsibilities and things, that was unsustainable. One or two people alone cannot take on a project like this; you have to get friends and comrades on board until you have the capacity to do what you need and use the different skills that you all have. For example, my background is in social media and so I knew how to build a social media following before we had really done anything, and that meant that we had an audience that was enthusiastic about crowdfunding us. I used my skills to make that happen. But we didn't have skills in renovating a building, so that took forever because we didn't know what we were doing, and it was slow and expensive.

So it's not just, oh, anyone can do it. It's hard. And you have to know how to manage your energy, and the resources that you have, and the skills that you have, to the best of your ability because you're going to fail in lots of—hopefully small—ways, and you have to pick yourself up from those and keep going.

We also thought about it for fucking ages before we did it, so we were dedicated to the idea before we started, and that was helpful as well. And we had a good pulse on what our community needs, which is important; you have to know what need you're fulfilling. We knew that our local community's needs were for free food, an alcohol-free queer space, an alcohol-free space that's open at night, a Jewish communal space outside shul [synagogue], and any space that is wheelchair accessible at all. Because when we first started, there were no accessible bathrooms on the whole of Victoria Road, or in this whole neighborhood. We were the first one, and now there are two—the place right next door to us has one now too, but I think that's it. So those were the biggest needs. And then internationally, having an anti-Zionist Jewish space was a need and having a Yiddish space was clearly a need. Know what needs you want to fulfill, and work out what your capacity is to meet those needs. And do what you can.

If what you can do is small, then do the small thing; don't do nothing. You can always make it bigger later. Don't let being daunted stop you.

❧   ❧   ❧

Moishe Holleb | בעלאָה השמ is a queer and trans Yiddish anarchist who cares a lot about food justice, Yiddish, supporting survivors of sexual violence, and trans health care. He recently moved to Brooklyn to be around more queer lefty Jews. His Instagram is @mishaholleb.

Alice Ross | עדיירפֿ לדייא is motivated by curiosity, unafraid of sincerity, and thinks you should make time to look at the moon. She is on Instagram as @sketchyalice and part of @leithfoodnotbombs.

The Pink Peacock collective included around forty different people over its three years of operation. Every one of them contributed to the space with their unique skills and insights, fostering community with their labor and dedication, building אבה םלועה (h'oylom h'bo, or the world to come).

# SOLIDARITY APOTHECARY: RECLAIMING LIFE

/

NICOLE ROSE

Just traveling home from seeing Kevan in [Her Majesty's Prison] Belmarsh. The only comfort of the day other than holding his hands was seeing all of my plant friends outside. It felt moving that nearly all the herbs featured in *The Prisoner's Herbal* book were [not only] a stone's throw away from the prison [but also that] they were all on the inside.

—Solidarity Apothecary, Instagram, March 1, 2022

As an anarchist and herbalist, I focus on supporting people experiencing state violence. This is the heartbeat of my work in the world.

For me, anarchism is the commitment to eradicating all forms of domination. I believe in a world without cages. I believe in collective care, self-determination, and responsibility to each other as well as the land. I am continuously inspired by movements, revolutionaries, and organizers around the globe, especially Black and Brown feminists and abolitionists who share frameworks of healing justice, abolition, mutual aid, and liberation. My goal as an herbalist is to contribute to developing health care infrastructure that builds autonomy beyond the state, capitalism, white supremacy, and patriarchy.

My love of plants was cultivated in prison, which for better or worse, has shaped my adult life. I've been supporting partners, friends, and comrades in prison for the last 17 years. I did a 3.5-year sentence myself after a huge wave of state repression against a campaign to close down Europe's largest animal testing company. Plants sustained me through that time, and many years later I wrote *The Prisoner's Herbal* book, which is distributed to prisoners worldwide. I now run a mutual aid project called the Solidarity Apothecary that focuses on working with plant medicines to support people experiencing state violence and am part of another mutual aid effort, Mobile Herbal Clinic Calais.

Having burned out, hard, writing about it, and eventually "recovering" (a complex and imperfect term), I also support organizers going through similar cycles of loss, despair, and overwhelm. Plant medicines offered me a path through the maze. And now with clinical training and huge amounts of learning from others doing this work, I'm able to offer the balm and comfort of plant medicines to others too. I send care packages to sites of resistance such as protest camps and offer one-to-one aid, recognizing that the front line is everywhere that we are doing the challenging work of struggling for freedom.

Until anarchists and other people committed to social change give radical attention to how we care for each other, we will always burn out, we will always feel unsupported, and thus we will remain dependent for "care" on state institutions that dehumanize us. Withdrawal is not an option, but transformation is.

## STATE VIOLENCE AND THE BODY

[Saw] my girl Sam at [Her Majesty's Prison] Eastwood Park. ... Her cancer is back. ... The prison has FAILED to even take her to [the] fucking hospital for her biopsies. ... [It] failed to take her to her pre-op appointment, so now the surgery that was meant to happen months ago has been pushed back AGAIN.

It's a really long story of ongoing neglect and harm. ...
She is lucky to still be fucking alive.

—Solidarity Apothecary, Instagram, March 19, 2022

State violence shapes people 's bodies. In prison, we referred
to health care as "health scare." It was such a dehumanizing
process to submit a written application to see a doctor, wait
for weeks, and then just be dismissed, patronized, or put
down during the two-minute consultation. Medical neglect
is the norm. My friend, for instance, nearly died of cancer in
prison after the authorities failed on nine separate occasions
to take her to hospital appointments for the lifesaving surgery
she needed. To cite just one statistic, in the United Kingdom,
the average age of death for those in prison is 56 years
compared to the wider UK expectancy of 81 years.[1] In the
United States, research has shown that this impact extends
to prisoners' families too. Life expectancy is 2.6 years shorter
for people who have an incarcerated or formerly incarcerated
family member than for those who don't.[2]

The relentless roller coaster of prisoner support also
impacts prisoners' families along with those organizers trying
their best to offer solidarity to incarcerated people so that they
can survive in unimaginable conditions. Those on the outside
often experience burnout, becoming physically exhausted,

1. Tumbi Otudeko, "Mind the Gap: Healthcare Disparities in UK
Prisons," Medact, August 21, 2020, https://medact.org/2020/blogs/
mind-the-gap-healthcare-disparities-in-uk-prisons/.

2. Emily Widra, "New Data: People with Incarcerated Loved Ones
Have Shorter Life Expectancies and Poorer Health," Prison Policy
Initiative, July 12, 2021, https://prisonpolicy.org/blog/2021/07/12/
family-incarceration/.

emotionally overwhelmed, and vicariously traumatized after years of prison visits, not to mention the chronic stress of being separated from people they love.

I've met hundreds of ex-prisoners, prisoners' families, and comrades across the world engaged in prisoner support work. Most don't come out of prison or this work unchanged. I'm not sure where I first heard the saying or from whom, but it has always stayed with me: "You can never really leave prison because prison never really leaves you." A framework related to "post-incarceration syndrome" is slowly emerging and increasingly being studied, yet it's still not clinically recognized despite thousands of prisoners living with complex post-traumatic stress from their captivity.

## HEALING AS LIBERATION

> Collecting hawthorn berries on my lunch break. They are one of my most beloved medicines, which I use in blends to support defendants experiencing repression. They strengthen the physical and emotional heart in so many ways, ... and are an amazing plant medicine for frontline organizers with heavy hearts.
>
> —Solidarity Apothecary, Instagram, September 24, 2020

Hypervigilance, muscle pain, nightmares, digestive issues, chronic inflammation, and on and on—the body doesn't lie about the effects of state violence, even if we hide our feelings behind movement machismo. What I learned studying herbalism, though, is that we can heal tissues, calm nervous systems, and attend to wounds of all kinds. Plant medicines offer us tools to survive and recover from state violence. They can help us move into different states of being through their direct effect on us, supporting us to shift many forms of chronic illness and so much more. Beyond just "consuming" herbs in a medicinal format, connecting with plants on a practical level (being outside, gardening, making medicine, etc.) can aid us in achieving a parasympathetic nervous system state, aka "rest and digest," where our bodies get a chance to relax and recover. For people scarred by trauma, such as from seeing the worst in other human beings who keep them in their cages, plants offer companionship and trust in a way that only nonhumans can.

Integrative models blending allopathic frameworks (especially emergency care infrastructure) with traditional and holistic forms of medicine have served communities well for thousands of years. The radical beauty of plant medicines is that you don't need to navigate an authoritarian or state-mediated system to access them. Knowledge is shared orally across generations. Those separated from traditional herbal lineages due to colonialism, capitalism, and oppression, including being displaced from land, are relearning herbalism through apprenticeships, DIY study/experimentation, popular education, and skill sharing, all of which enables people to access the information they need to take care of themselves and each other.

Feminist health movements have focused on this for decades, with anarchistic feminists in particular seeing the connection between bodily autonomy and the expansive struggle for freedom in all realms of life. Emma Goldman, for instance, herself a nurse and midwife, took direct action to bring contraceptive devices into the United States and disseminate information on birth control and abortion at a time when both access and knowledge were illegal. She saw her feminist health practices as inseparable from her anarchist values and ideas.[3]

## SOLIDARITY APOTHECARY AS MUTUAL AID

In Poland at the herbal space, I met a Ukrainian woman who told me her and her husband make rose tincture from roses in their garden. I told her we have rose tincture and took it from the stack of drawers we have there, and she started to cry. No amount of tincture could take away the pain of leaving your husband [back home] to fight a Russian invasion. But I'm glad in that moment I could pass her something that showed her we cared, we are with her, and that rose is available to hold her tears through grief and rage and pain.

—Solidarity Apothecary, Instagram, May 25, 2022

The mission of the Solidarity Apothecary is to materially support revolutionary struggles and communities with plant medicines to strengthen collective autonomy, self-defense, and resilience, whether to climate change, capitalism, borders, or so much more. Anarchists have always been dedicated to

---

3. "Emma Goldman—Women's Rights—Birth Control," Jewish Women's Archive, accessed December 8, 2023, https://jwa.org/womenofvalor/goldman/womens-rights/birth-control.

mutual aid, such as smuggling food to prisoners and providing safe houses for people on the run from fascist regimes. The Solidarity Apothecary is herbal medicine as mutual aid.

The main focus of the Solidarity Apothecary is making and distributing plant medicines to people experiencing state violence and repression. This includes people being arrested, on trial, detained, imprisoned, or recovering from these experiences as well as prisoners' families, frontline organizers, and others. Herbal solidarity comes in the form of care packages or one-to-one support, or as part of our mobile clinic. A group may contact me asking for herbal support. We'll talk through any medications, and whether people are pregnant or have any potential risk factors that could contraindicate with herbs. I'll then prepare something that speaks to them and their group's needs.

One common need is nervous system support. Nervines—a group of plants that affect the nervous system—can help support our bodies to relax and gain respite from the intensity of the fight-flight-freeze response we feel when experiencing or reexperiencing trauma and stress. It might be a tea blend to help people sustain energy for difficult emotional meetings, or a blend to help people prevent or recover from burnout. Common nervines that I work with include rose (*Rosa* spp.), hawthorn flowers and berries (*Crataegus monogyna*), and lemon balm (*Melissa officinalis*). I tend to make glycerites, which are herbs infused in glycerine—a fantastic alternative to alcohol.

I may also send people general support for their immune systems through the mail, including a strong cough syrup, chest rub, and incredible immune tonic that brings together herbs such as thyme (*Thymus vulgaris*), ginger (*Zingiber officinale*), turmeric (*Curcuma longa*), echinacea (*Echinacea purpurea*), and elderberry (*Sambucus nigra*). Another favorite is fire cider vinegar—long revered in different folk herbalism traditions as a spicy immune enhancer to help people survive winters. I try extremely hard to make medicines from the land where I live and that I care for. If I'm unable to grow at the scale needed, I will source herbs from local organic suppliers, or a broader network of herb growers and foragers that support the Solidarity Apothecary.

It's not just the biological effects on our bodies, however; gifting medicine is an act of showing that we care about each other and see the violence someone is experiencing. In Bristol, many parents lost their children to prison following the March 2021 Kill the Bill riot, a response to a new, repressive policing bill in the United Kingdom and the murder of Sarah Everard by a police officer. Herbal medicines were commonly distributed after sentencing to these parents, who often became tearful just knowing that someone cares about them and even thought of this as a need. Lavender-infused oil (with olive oil from Palestine) is a favorite sleep aid for people experiencing grief and distress. Likewise, rose glycerite helps people "hold steady" amid turbulent times in their lives.

For me, anarchist organizing isn't about just helping prepare people for their trials or time in prison. It's not just sharing their addresses publicly to generate letters and fundraising to meet their material needs. It is also about expressing care— unlearning machismo, and actually talking about the effects of state violence on our bodies, relationships, and movements. And it's about recognizing that care and solidarity comes from nonhumans too; that plants can directly support us in surviving this world.

As an herbalist, I offer more in-depth, personalized support on a one-to-one basis as well. This involves a forty- to ninety-minute session exploring a person's full health history, creating unique herbal and nutritional recommendations, and aiding them with whichever medicine may best support them. This offering is shared at a sliding scale, from completely free for people without papers, people experiencing state violence, or those leaving prison, to more expensive packages for people with the financial resources to pay for my time and medicines, thereby redistributing their wealth to support others for whom it otherwise would be financially impossible to access this kind of in-depth care.

As an abolitionist, I cannot do this work without centering people in prison. When I walked out those gates, I knew I couldn't leave others behind. Even though a part of me never wanted to think about prison ever again, I also knew I couldn't accept the injustice, racism, and violence continuing. Until the last human and animal are out of prison, this will be my emphasis for the rest of my life. As it's nearly impossible to send in any kind of herbs or have consultations with people, the best thing we can do is to support people in prison to study herbalism themselves. That's why I created the The Prisoner's Herbal; it is written for people in prison who want to learn about the medicinal properties of plants commonly found in prison courtyards. Among other information, it contains ten detailed plant profiles as well as instructions on how to prepare plant medicines in prison. The book is based on my experience of using herbs throughout my own prison sentence.

More than two thousand copies have been sent to prisoners via different prisoner books and support projects, and we now have a dedicated crew called the Prisoner Herbalism Collective that makes it all happen. Our collective meets monthly, and between us all, we coordinate sending books to prisoners in the United Kingdom, United States, and Mexico. In September 2022, *The Prisoner's Herbal* was translated into Spanish. We've created two editions of this version of the book: one for people imprisoned in the Spanish state, and the other for people incarcerated across Abya Yala, the name in Guna for the so-called Americas, used by millions of Indigenous peoples across these continents. *La Herbolaria de lxs Presxs* has now gone to prisoners in Mexico, Chile, and farther afield in Immigration and Customs Enforcement centers and prisons in the United States. The launch event in Mexico was hosted at the Plantón de Mujeres Mazatecas, a site of ongoing occupation by Mazatec women family members of the political prisoners in Eloxochitlán de Flores Magón, Oaxaca. This fierce feminist campaign connects the intimate, personal pain of loved ones being imprisoned with oppression and injustice worldwide. This for me encapsulates anarchist feminism: the emotional, relational, and animist reality embedded in acts of care and resistance; the personal and political along with the refusal to separate the two; and keen insights into gendered oppression while refusing to be reductionist and instead always seeing the interconnectedness.

In addition, many prisoners are now undertaking distance learning courses in prison with our support. Every letter I open from someone inside nearly always makes me cry. People write to us saying how much the book has inspired them. To connect with plants in prison is life changing. With relationship and connection, we are never alone. As just one example, a prisoner wrote,

> I love your herbal book. ... Personally I cannot overstate how this book has helped me in prison. I have many ailments from asthma, COPD, [and] severe reactive skin. Unfortunately our prison yard is mostly concrete. But I have managed to treat my ailments by picking dandelion leaves to eat and wash. Also we have some plantain that grows so I use that for lots of things. Also we have a bit of clover so I use all [of] what I can. On the out[side], I lived in a field and never touched detergent. I have a good knowledge of herbs, but your book has bolstered up my own knowledge, and the use of canteen items as well is amazing. Thank you all so much for this book. Herbs keep me alive in prison, and give me light and greenery.

## MOBILE HERBAL CLINIC CALAIS

Another week in Calais and Dunkirk [amid makeshift encampments for those who survived the journey from France across the Channel to England] with the Mobile Herbal Clinic Calais. ... With worsening weather, people are making more desperate and dangerous attempts to cross the border. We met more than one person who had developed serious flu from being in cold water trying to cross in a boat. People had broken hands from trying to jump fences and climb under lorries. ... We gave out more medicine than ever, and many people came back asking for refills of cough syrup.

—Solidarity Apothecary, Instagram, November 2019

It needs no introduction that state violence is racialized, classed, and gendered in its design and application. The British border is no exception. People arrive in northern France after having traveled for months and thousands of miles in order to then cross the Channel to apply for asylum in the United Kingdom. Many have come from Syria, Kurdistan, Afghanistan, Iran, Sudan, and Eritrea, to name a few places. Their journeys expose the horror of white supremacy in what's often dubbed Fortress Europe. In Calais, people live in outdoor encampments with constant police evictions and brutality as well as food and water insecurity after having already faced a dangerous trek of crossings via water or hidden in trucks—both of which have taken many lives.

For the last five years, Mobile Herbal Clinic Calais has maintained a presence in northern France supporting refugees and migrants risking their lives to cross the British border. I regularly visit Calais most months as a field coordinator and herbal first aider being mentored by senior herbalists and doctors on our team. Since October 2019, we have seen more than five thousand people with upper respiratory conditions, skin complaints, digestive issues, and more, not to mention injuries inflicted by the police. Our medicines are crafted by a dedicated network of grassroots medicine makers and growers, with expenses covered by do-it-ourselves fundraisers. During the first months of the pandemic, we made and distributed more than six thousand medicines in fifteen hundred packs, crossing the Channel regularly despite restrictions. Each pack included cough syrup, antimicrobial vinegar, salt water, and a chest rub to alleviate COVID-19 symptoms. We also included a leaflet in five languages about where and how to access further health care during the pandemic.

At times, it can literally feel like a "sticking plaster," as we say in England, when you're applying bandages or engaged in wound care. Yet it's clear after thousands of conversations that the solidarity is valued and needed, and people feel warmth and affinity toward the medicines we used, particularly because many of the travelers are coming from countries with strong herbal medicine traditions.

Herbal medicine comes into its own in response to upper respiratory infections (coughs, colds, flu, sinus infections, etc.). We give people cough syrup, immune tonic, chest rubs, salt water, lozenges, and so on, to help shift their symptoms. We listen to people's chests if they've been coughing for longer than a week, and refer them for antibiotics or a hospital when needed. Our work in the region is not just about symptomatic relief; our multimodality team of doctors, paramedics, and herbalists aims to find those people who may slip through the net and yet need urgent care. One man I met who'd had a long-term cough and sore throat actually had tuberculosis. He was able to access urgent care during a two-week hospital stay, and it was amazing to shake his hand on the next visit once he was out of the hospital. We also offer bruise ointments and heat packs for people with long-term musculoskeletal injuries that flare up when they're walking massive amounts of miles every day. And we've distributed garlic, ginger, and lemons as general immune support for folks to cook with in their informal encampments.

In Calais and Dunkirk, there is a constant flow of new arrivals, so we give them a guide to all the services in the area (produced and translated into multiple languages by a group called Refugee Infobus). Many people are not aware that health care is possible if you do not have papers or money. The reviews of La Pass, the local free clinic, are mixed; many report experiences of racism and frustration, though others have had a more positive experience. Either way, it's important to know that the clinic exists and is available if people need it.

Still, many people won't take the long bus ride to the clinic, especially due to racism risks, and so working in the camps is essential. Many people have secondary infected wounds, such as a small mosquito bite that's become infected. We use conventional first aid dressings, but will often bring in herbal tools such as baikal skullcap (*Scutellaria baicalensis*) powder combined with aloe vera gel into a paste. People will look at you wondering what the hell are you putting on them, only to come back over the following days delighted that their stubborn wound is finally healing.

We've had so many beautiful and tender conversations about people's experience with herbal medicine where they are coming from too. It's a validating reminder that herbal medicine is the primary form of health care for most people on the planet, and not everywhere has the prejudices and reductionist attitudes toward herbal remedies that is prevalent in the United Kingdom, where many people have been separated from the land for seven generations of industrialization, and influenced by "Enlightenment" era notions that separate people from their bodies and landscapes.

## CARE IS A RADICAL ACT

> I've had this tiny anxiety in the back of my head that people wouldn't find [our humble herbal medicine] useful in this context. Like WTF can some herb tea do right now? But the demand has taken me aback, and everyone is constantly saying how needed and appreciated it is.
>
> —Solidarity Apothecary, Instagram, November 2019

Plant medicines gave me the opportunity to see that our work for liberation is not just about social war but also about healing. Indeed, developing and experimenting with collective, transformational ways to heal actually *is* the work. In an abolitionist context, this can mean searching for forms of healing that don't involve reimprisonment or further state violence (such as being sent to a psychiatric hospital). It can and should involve recognizing that abolitionist work is as much about trauma recovery as it is about resistance—that reclaiming life from trauma is resistance. Recovery must be a politicized practice and collective endeavor. It can mean engaging in methods of healing that build mutual aid and reconnection, solidarity and social relationships.

Care is a radical act, and one of our biggest weapons. Collective care points beyond all the structures we fight against while simultaneously already embodying the alternatives we fight and yearn for. Yet for too long, the centrality of care to life itself has been downplayed or erased, including within anarchist circles. Anarcha-feminists have challenged the invisibilization of care, even as they've typically been the ones to engage in the myriad types of "care work" that form the backbone of anarchist infrastructure, and are essential to everything that anarchists believe in and practice.

Plants sustain life too, despite the fact that "we" in the colonized Western world have been taught to no longer see plants, much less have a relationship with them. Yet as Indigenous writer and scientist Robin Wall Kimmerer observes, "In some Native languages the term for plants translates to 'those who take care of us.'"[4] Plants take care of each other and their ecosystems, including taking care of us. They take care of us in prison courtyards and refugee camps, when fleeing war zones or working toward a world free of domination, exploitation, and oppression. The Solidarity Apothecary and my related projects are just tiny conduits; the herbs themselves are mutual aid.

❀ ❀ ❀

---

4. Robin Wall Kimmerer, *Braiding Sweetgrass: Indigenous Wisdom, Scientific Knowledge, and the Teachings of Plants* (Minneapolis: Milkweed Editions, 2013), 229.

Nicole Rose (she/her) is an anarchist organizer and herbalist living in England who has been active in struggles for human, animal, and earth liberation for over twenty years. She is also the author of *The Prisoner's Herbal*, *Overcoming Burnout*, and *The Medicinal Herb Colouring Book*. You can find all of her work at www.solidarityapothecary.org and @solidarity.apothecary on Instagram.

# NORTH STAR HEALTH COLLECTIVE: TENDING TO THE SPARKS

/

MAGS BEALL
AND CORY MARIA DACK

**Mags:** It's the last few days of May 2020. Or maybe it's the first few days of June. I don't really know anymore. I haven't slept significantly since May 26, the day after the murder of George Floyd. He was assassinated at Thirty-Eighth Street and Chicago Avenue—a place that would become known (and still is) as George Floyd Square. In the days immediately following his killing, the Third Precinct of the Minneapolis Police Department at Lake Street and Minnehaha Avenue was the site of a pitched battle that ended in police fleeing and the building being set on fire. The structure is still a fenced-off, charred shell as of this writing over three years later. The house I lived in at the time was—as the crow flies—halfway between those two intersections.

There is no way here to capture the days and weeks of that time in Minneapolis, in my neighborhood. The beauty, fear, and complexities, or even just the sounds. And for anyone unfamiliar with this city, it may have seemed like a random spark—this death. It wasn't. For years, the murder of Black, Indigenous, and Brown people here has been at epidemic levels. This moment was only one culmination, among others, of years of struggle. I would never claim to have been at the center of any of that. I played a support role, predominantly as a street medic with North Star Health Collective. Yet what happened was a rebellion, an exploding ecosystem of glorious rage, solidarity, and care in which we were all fighting like hell for a new and different Minneapolis and world.

❖　❖　❖

**Cory:** I was vetted by North Star about forty-eight hours after the community burned the Third Precinct to the ground. Less than a week earlier, I'd returned to the United States the night before George Floyd was murdered, after spending seventy days in a military lockdown in Ecuador at the start of the pandemic. Knowing that it lacked the resources to handle the assault of COVID-19 that we were seeing in Europe at that time, and with only thirty-seven confirmed cases in the country, Ecuador put a strict nationwide curfew into place that ran from 2:00 p.m. to 6:00 a.m. each day.

At 2:00 p.m., sirens blared all over Quito, the capital city where I was then living, and at 2:30 p.m. helicopters could be seen flying overhead, making sure that people were in fact inside for the rest of the day and night. The consequences for breaking curfew and other regulations involved being fined a month's salary and thrown into jail for three to four months. Having come from this extreme Ecuadorian lockdown, I was still in the mindset of taking curfews seriously. Early on in the George Floyd uprising, and shortly after curfews were being set in both Minneapolis and Saint Paul, I heard a rumor that street medics were allowed "curfew immunity." This turned out to be a laughable fallacy, yet as I like to say, "I came for the lie; I stayed for the community."

Although there is absolutely no such thing as curfew immunity for street medics, I'm glad this false rumor led me to a phone call that changed my life. With my hands shaking out of nervousness, I called a number given to me by a friend of a friend and left a voicemail with someone at North Star Health Collective, asking if I could become a street medic. As a certified Wilderness First Responder for over twelve years at that point, I had already put together a makeshift med kit and was carrying it around with me at the daily protests. I felt like providing medical and emotional care was something that I could do for my communities during this time of crisis. Back in 2016, I had received some basic street medic training while at Standing Rock, but the early days of the George Floyd uprising were where I first saw frontline duty. Connecting with North Star gave me a community that was incredibly supportive and empowering.

Before long, running as a street medic was what I did with my life for the rest of 2020, and have done ever since.

❧　❧　❧

North Star Health Collective "ran"—shorthand for going out as a street medic—in support of what would become known as "the uprising." Later, it was called the first uprising or George Floyd uprising because of the one that was kicked off the following year by another murder-by-police, this time of Daunte Wright. We ran beginning with the first march after George Floyd was killed, although we had no idea what was coming at the end of that march when it reached the Third Precinct. As the anger on the streets found traction and sustained itself beyond a day or two, or even a few, North Star wasn't fully prepared for the level of labor to come in caring for our communities.

This is not an attempt to tell that story, even though we'll reference it. Instead, it is a reflection on *how*, as medics, we engage in movements and grassroots organizing, because the voluntary, self-organized practice of offering health care on the streets is often overlooked when we focus on our most intense moments or the ones that are usually centered in the media spotlight. That *how* is also the way by which we have come through the uprising(s) stronger.

## A BRIEF HISTORY

How we were drawn to this work is unique to each of our lived experiences, of course, but the street medic world has a long and powerful history. We usually start the story in the civil rights era—though there are lineages far older than that—and share the origins of the Medical Committee for Human Rights, which had a protest arm that took care of people in the streets in places like Selma, Alabama. We honor the health care work of the Black Panther Party and Young Lords.[1] The teachers of the next generation of street medics came from that time and taught those of us in the "another world is possible" era in the late 1990s and early 2000s the same skills. Medic skills evolved and continue to do so to this day, when now those of us from that earlier time in turn teach the new generation. North Star's tale falls into these last chapters.

North Star Health Collective was founded in 2008 in preparation for the Republican National Convention set to be hosted in Saint Paul that year. Founding member

1. For more on this history, see, for example, "Medical Committee for Human Rights," SNCC Digital, accessed December 8, 2023, https://snccdigital.org/inside-sncc/alliances-relationships/mchr/; Johanna Fernández, *The Young Lords: A Radical History* (Chapel Hill: University of North Carolina Press, 2020); Alondra Nelson, *Body and Soul: The Black Panther Party and the Fight against Medical Discrimination* (Minneapolis: University of Minnesota Press, 2013).

Kat Donnelly notes that "2008 was a really intense time in Minneapolis organizing ... and we got hit real hard by repression. Real hard. A lot of people got very, very hurt." North Star wasn't an exception, and so while we were medics for that large action, there was a good bit of care work that was needed for the community and ourselves afterward. This work wove its way through the following years, through Occupy and other encampments, supporting protests in the region such as against a NATO summit in Chicago in 2012, and during the 2014 uprising in Ferguson, Missouri, after police murdered Mike Brown. Here in Minneapolis, between the ongoing killing of Black people by cops and responses to the rise of the alt-right, we were consistently doing what we could to support struggles. Then in 2019, "Donald Trump came to town. And then the pandemic happened. And then George Floyd was killed. ... And then we've been just running flat-out for the last two years," says Kat. And when we weren't running, we were leading trainings.

What came with the uprising was more than just that "flat-out" run. It meant that we had to change how we did things. In some ways, everything changed after the murder of George Floyd, but what carried us through and continues to do so is that we never lost sight of our values. In unparalleled experiences of upheaval across whole swaths of the Twin Cities, we were able to breathe and ask ourselves, "OK, how do we participate yet stay grounded in who we are?" Before May 25, 2020, when a protest happened, the core organizers—a loosely affiliated group of medics that chose to do more of the logistical organizing—would reach out to all the trained medics, including ourselves, to see who could go run. Maybe someone dispatched from afar, but there was not much of a structure; we hadn't needed one. By three days into the George Floyd uprising, we realized that we needed to build something more solid. Our existing medics were already burning out from the intensity on the streets, while people wanting to street medic were coming out of the woodwork. These new folks were excited by what was happening around them, and some had medical training, yet the majority of them were almost entirely without street medic training and sometimes any medical training at all.

While this is a brief glance at our history, much of what North Star was able to hold during the uprising and into the present is based on years of developing our theories and practices, and building out our ideas, trainings, and what is at the heart of our work. This can't be understated. A moment of uprising can turn the world upside down, but our practices can carry us through those moments well (or not) regardless of our role. North Star and street medics in general, along with many other roles integral to this fight, cannot be seen or understood only in moments of upheaval or crisis, because how we act in those moments is defined by much longer, deeper relational work.

## NORTH STAR ETHICS

There is a difference between being a street medic and being a medic-in-the-streets. Health care professionals who hit the streets with their med bags are not necessarily prepared to give care to people under extreme duress with limited resources. And unless you're a trained street medic, you might not be operating with the same values that North Star holds. We are there to serve our communities by giving consent-based care and spreading calm. We are the antithesis of the "Batmans" who charge into situations with their med kits and credentials in hand, more interested in playing the role of hero while forcing "care" onto patients than actually doing the deep work of decolonizing themselves or the medical systems that employ them. It's one thing to provide medical care to those wounded on the front lines. It's another to do so while making sure that the patient's bodily autonomy and dignity is prioritized.

When North Star trains community members—whether in basic health and safety or as full street medics—we start with our ethics. Our core values include consent, do no harm, take no shit, and noncooperation with state actors and fascists. North Star believes that in order to help keep people calm, slow is smooth and smooth is fast—meaning that we're more capable of moving through a situation quickly and respectfully if we slow down and remain calm. We maintain people's confidentiality and only work within our scope—that is, a set of skills that we've self-determined together make sense in our role as street medics. We rely on a buddy system and accountability, lean into flexibility, and support a diversity of tactics. These ethics map onto the anarchistic and feministic frameworks, among other liberatory ones, of the collective.

For us, it all starts with *consent*. Most of our medics remember the moment in training when one of us jumped up and down yelling "Consent! Consent! Consent!" over and over again. Consent is embedded in *everything* we aspire to do. It's rooted in both prefiguring the kinds of solidaristic care we ascribe to and aiming not to replicate the white Christian supremacist, misogynist culture of the dominant conventional medical system, which among other things, typically follows a hierarchical structure of "the doctor knows best" and imposes that onto people seen as "patients." Instead, as Kat puts it, North Star emphasizes "enthusiastic, radical consent. In every interaction, it's something that I strive for." We see our relationship to those we're aiding in the streets as both mutualistic and a way to "honor how we each move through the world," says Kat.

From this place of centering consent, we get to the notion of "do no harm." This is an ethic that supposedly runs through medical culture and yet we know how little that tracks with people's lived experiences. When we really take this seriously, it runs deep. Sometimes North Star is perceived as being overly cautious because of this value. As an example, we don't carry medication to give out—even over-the-counter meds like ibuprofen—because when we've never interacted with someone before, we don't know anything about them, such as their allergies or medical history. So if we're trying to challenge the ways that capitalism and patriarchy push things onto people, or that as health care providers, we somehow know better than you about your own body, then in a brief instance on the street, we can't pretend that we know what will or will not harm you.

Furthermore, this gets at a demilitarized approach. As we mentioned, "medics" poured into town during the uprising, with some asserting, "I was a combat medic in the military," and bringing along an attitude of "I'm the big man who can throw someone over my shoulder and run them out of the fray." In the streets—in a time of resistance—this looks exactly like the shit so many of us femme, **BIPOC**, queer, and trans folks experience in the dominant system of medicine. We reject such practices so as to shift the experience for both the person offering and the person accepting care. Parvaneh, a newer medic, underscored "just how blatantly fucked up the medical system is" and that North Star continually stresses that fact "through all the trainings. There's a super deep understanding of how fucking colonial, racist, sexist, and homophobic the medical system is, and how we need to consistently be pushing against that as medics. Unlearning that is so active."

Street medics love to say, more expansively, "Do no harm. Take no shit." This encompasses our core value of doing no harm, but is also shorthand for not being neutral. We don't work with the state; we don't work with fascists. We're on a side, and we show up so that our side can keep fighting. For example, if you take a standard **CPR** class, you'll be taught to call 911 as a core part of any response. In North Star, we learn how to recognize when someone needs higher medical care, get consent from them before engaging with 911 or emergency medical services (EMS), and not give away sensitive or identifying information to emergency services. We center not only the person we're caring for and act as an advocate for them if they desire but recognize that we are in an antagonistic relationship with the state too. When the EMS and police show up, we don't chat with them like we're buddies just because we might have similar training. We don't cooperate with or even ever talk to them unless it is explicitly in an advocacy role and with the injured person's consent.

Jay, who has run with North Star, notes that these ethics

are for them about "moving through the world with a radical attention to how I impact other people, and doing that in a way that doesn't devalue myself. I feel like those are often two things in our culture; we have a hard time balancing or even acknowledging our impact and caring for ourselves."

❖ ❖ ❖

**Mags:** When I think about why I'm a street medic, I think about an experience the first night of the uprising after the murder of George Floyd. People weren't particularly prepared for it to turn into such a street battle. The cops were in hard defense of their precinct; it had been breached and was surrounded on three sides. They were firing tear gas every way they could. They would fire a round, and people would move back to let the chemical spray pass. And there, in that moment, is my medic buddy and me. We wash peoples' eyes out so that they can advance again. Twenty years ago it was the same. We wash your eyes or tend to your wounds so that you can keep fighting.

❖ ❖ ❖

**Cory:** After Trump lost the 2020 presidential election, his supporters began to hold regular protests in front of the governor's mansion in Saint Paul. Counterprotesters would show up, often resulting in clashes between the two groups. A police presence was constant at these events. One such Saturday, my buddy and I arrived on-site and were quickly approached by two people marked as medics who we'd never seen before. Dressed head to toe in camouflage and with the familiar posture of someone who is obviously taking themselves too seriously, one of these so-called medics introduced themselves and proceeded to tell us about an alleged protocol we were supposed to follow for calling ambulances. North Star's protocol is to only call an ambulance with patient consent. In sharp contrast, it was clear that this "medic" believed they had the authority to call an ambulance whether their patient wanted them to or not.

With the colonizing air of a white person who is used to deciding who is in charge and who is not, this person bowled forward, "And don't forget, you *have* to treat *anyone* who gets hurt today, including any cops or fascists! You have a *moral* and *legal* obligation to do this. And if you don't want to follow your *moral* and *legal* obligations, then what are you even doing here?" The "medic" locked eyes with me as if I had outwardly shuddered at the thought of treating a cop or fascist. I know that I had not, in fact, reacted at all; as a woman of color, I have had a lot of practice keeping my face and body language neutral while a white person lectures me or bosses me around with an assumed authority that they don't actually have. I wait for them to finish having their moment and then walk away, continuing to live my life how I see fit. In this particular instance, I knew that I wasn't bound to the so-called ethics that a random medic-in-the-street had suddenly sprung on us.

I wouldn't have given the interaction that much more thought except that my buddy was pretty shaken up by it, initially worried that we needed to do what the medic-in-the-street told us. "We don't need to listen to random people whose values seem super suspicious," I assured my buddy. "We get to hold to our values." To validate my instincts, I called our dispatcher to explain what had happened. She was horrified that the other medic had tried to pressure us to put ourselves in danger by treating a cop or fascist. "Absolutely not!" I can still hear our dispatcher's voice in my head, booming out of the speaker on my phone as my buddy and I huddled around it in the cool November air. "There actually is *no* moral or legal obligation to treat cops or fascists, *especially* not as a BIPOC person; that could really put you in danger!" I remember feeling really grateful that after six months of running nonstop as a North Star medic, I was grounded in our collective's ethics, which helped me see through the bullshit, and make a better decision for myself, my buddy, and the people we were there to protect. Ignoring that shitty white medic's oppressive and obsessive need to assert dominance and control is one of the ways I really leaned into the "take no shit" part of "do not harm, take no shit."

## NORTH STAR PRACTICES

Holding a set of anarchist values while in motion is important. North Star often thrives—or knows why we're not—because of our practices. We work to live this out in everything we do. Which means that we develop protocols as well as discuss how to evolve and change, but from a strong rooting in what we are working to build. It's granular, like when we check in with each other at the start of an action. It guides us, such that we insist on never running alone. It's why we have a whole dispatch system so as to care for each other on, and as we're leaving, the streets. Our ethics supply us with a compass for the wide-ranging and challenging ongoing process of remaking care work in the world today.

## BUDDIES AND THE RITUAL OF OUR CHECK-INS

To understand our check-ins, you have to understand that we always run with at least one other person and sometimes more. If there are three medics at a march, they all stick together. If there are more, they can split into pairs or trios. The larger collective trusts the autonomy of the medics on the ground to decide how to do that within our protocols. Buddies are important for several reasons—safety, support, accountability, and just plain logistics, to name a few. When we train street medics, before we ever get to medical skills, we teach our ethics and then our buddy system because it is a key practice of those ethics. In each training, we teach and stress PEARLY (*p*hysical vulnerabilities, *e*motional vulnerabilities, *a*rrestability, *r*ole, *l*oose ends, and *y*es [or no] to buddying), and buddy pairs go through this list with each other at the start of a run.

Whether we're approaching a candlelight vigil or thousand-person march, check-ins give us a moment to ground ourselves, within ourselves and to one another. We do this even if we have the pleasure of running as a street medic with several of our best friends—friends who've been in our lives for years before we ever became street medics. PEARLY allows us room to be dynamic human beings, capable of changing our boundaries as needed every time we run. There's also a sort of secular holiness in practicing this ritual. It prepares and calms us the way that reverence prepares and calms a person in a moment of spirituality. This is unsurprising, as caring for our communities is a holy and sacred act.

"It's a ritual that it allows us to also do something really important, which is acknowledge vulnerability and fear. And I feel like my fear is most dangerous to me and others when it's left untended and unnoticed," explains Jay, adding,

> How am I vulnerable? What things will break if I don't hold them or if I'm not here to hold them? What do you need to know about my body to keep me safe from really intense harm? You can't really do PEARLY without noticing what makes you afraid. And I feel like going through that with somebody else is the only way to not be ashamed about it, otherwise I'm going to do something stupid in a dangerous situation to try to prove I'm not afraid. When we do PEARLY at the beginning, we're writing our own story about what it means to do something dangerous and what it means to be afraid and where our values live in those choices, as opposed to capitalism's values or from our fucking martyrdom complexes. There's nothing more radical than to say to your buddy, "I've never spent close time with you, but our work is now to keep each other safe."

## DISPATCH

Buddies on the ground are backed up by our dispatchers, who offer care as well, but remotely. Our dispatch is a support system made up of people who are away from the action and can keep tabs for the medics on big-picture information, such as what's being reported on trusted live streams or Signal threads—say, about where the cops are or where there's a serious injury. Dispatchers can also respond to questions about protocols or where extra medic supplies are located. Most important, dispatchers know where medics are at all times when they're running, who each medic wants as their emergency contact in case they are arrested or hurt on the street, and that each medic has gotten in and out of the action safely. Historically, North Star had a loose way of doing dispatch, but during the first days of the uprising, we built a complex system involving Signal threads, encrypted spreadsheets, and dispatching protocols, allowing friends and then other vetted folks to do dispatch from within and far beyond Minneapolis.

North Star sees dispatch as a duty to our medics and never a burden. Our commitment to our medics is to know where and how they are. To care for each other is to take responsibility for each other. In numerous actions across the continent, for example, street medics have been targeted by both police and fascists. Dispatchers share such intel with our medics, and let them decide whether they want to keep running that night or not, and where. If the medic wants to be taken off the streets, dispatchers help them do so as safely as possible. We then make sure that the remaining medics have buddies, including by activating on-call medics. Dispatch might feel overbearing to some medics, as in, for instance, "Why do we have to remember to check out when we leave?" But we see it as working to solidify a culture of collective care by holding everyone through each action.

For us, building and holding such structures, such agreements and protocols, is part and parcel of the active work of building the world we want in the shell of the old. Many of us are in the medical field, or have some relationship to it as part of our jobs, history, or future. We reckon with the myriad problems of those institutions daily. So when we borrow some skills from "our day jobs" to apply in the streets, we choose to craft something else in that self-organized space; we aspire to practice and prefigure other ways of doing care work. That means that as a collective, we're continually trying to balance our knowledge and humility, our protocols and flexibility—which is both messy and risky as well as beautiful. Jay captures that generative balance:

> What really drew me into North Star was this way to create boundaries, love and care, and ethical support and structures around providing care work that held me accountable to the people I was caring for, and protected me in relationship with others as well. I was desperate to find a way to be a carer in the world that didn't just destroy me. And I also was so deeply moved and connected to what I think is like a deep and anarchist core principle as well: that everybody has agency, and my "job" as a medic isn't to decide things for people; it's to take care of them and support them in making the choices that they need to take care of themselves. In Judaism, there's a concept called *halacha*, which is often translated as law, but it literally means the way of going. And the ethos behind being a North Star street medic feels like halacha—together

we are finding a way of going. I found other parts of my life suddenly shifting in relationship to those principles and ideals.

## A FULL DIVERSITY OF TACTICS

It's easy to look at the past few years and focus on the burned buildings and pitched street battles. We can't see those times clearly here without that; the charred remains of a police precinct stand on one side of South Minneapolis with an intact yet still protected precinct, encircled by barricades and barbed wire, sitting on the other end of Lake Street. Street medics show up when needed. We do so without judgment of tactics or a role in deciding them. That means that we don't just treat your burns from a tear gas canister; we stick by those who need to express themselves in many ways.

Frequently "a diversity of tactics" gets used as a code that it has to be OK to burn things down. But what the twenty-four-hour social media cycle probably missed is that in the years during, following, and in between uprisings, there have been marches, protests, community assemblies, vigils, communal mourning, building occupations, mutual aid efforts, and more. We don't, as medics, have endless capacity or time, and so we can only do so much and hope that others fill in the gaps. Still, we aren't just there for the fire. As individuals, we have many different feelings about various tactics being used at different points and in different places. As a collective, we try to show up where we are invited and needed, because people who are organizing and agitating can use care.

What we strive for is to be a group that makes the best tactics and strategies possible—*because* people are cared for.

We don't have set rules, just living questions that we ask ourselves, such as, What is the definition of the streets? Those types of questions allow Autumn, as a street medic,

> to connect and be vulnerable. Which I feel is different than being out and being like, fuck the system! *Fuck the system!* I definitely feel and love to participate in that. But I think of the experience of, say, the small march where I was positioned right by Daunte Wright's mom. The sentencing [for the killer] had just come out, and as we were calling out the names [of Daunte and so many others murdered by police], there was so much fucking grief. As a medic, I was able to be soft in that moment and just feel that grief with Daunte's mom as people were naming off the names, repeating back who was murdered, who was lynched, and yelling her kid's name. I'm super grateful we're all here for such times, because Daunte's mom needed to be at that modern-day funeral procession.

That day, in that anger and grief, someone was clearly upset, yelling and moving around erratically. As street medics, we didn't interrupt or stop that person. We let them be in their rage yet also stayed close in case they needed support. To street medic shouldn't be an interruption of legitimate emotional response but rather a means of holding people during it.

## CARING FOR THE CARERS

Of course, this doesn't ever come easy or with some magical clarity. Many of us are burned out right now, even though much of our work isn't happening during intense street battles. Much of our work is actually preventative—offering sunscreen and electrolytes-type stuff. But it's almost as if we've been on call for over three years since the uprising. So we've had to wrestle with what it is to care for ourselves as well. Jay observes that

> we can be so thoughtful and so careful about how we connect and move through the world, and also not destroy ourselves in that process. Everybody gets to say yes or no to anything that's happening. And if I really believe in that [consent] for other people, I have to believe that about myself, because I notice that the moments I don't believe that about myself are the moments I start stepping over other people's consent and agency. When we care for ourselves it's disruptive of a story that's so convenient to capitalism, which is that people just care and then die, right? They don't get to keep growing. I don't think until I really encountered and tried to live out that principle that I actually understood that capitalism wins when caretakers die and burnout. It had never occurred to me that there was another way.

North Star has made it our business to *not* allow this to happen to our medics. A clear example is when eleven of us were arrested on November 4, 2020, the day after the US presidential elections. In what became known as "the most expensive dance party in the history of Minnesota," multiple law enforcement agencies kettled nearly seven hundred protesters who were in the process of marching off I-94, after having temporarily blocked it, back into residential neighborhoods. The police trapped protesters, medics, and independent media on the freeway for upward of five hours, and a dance party broke out to pass the time.[2] Immediately North Star demonstrated incredible care to the carers—from contacting our family members to let them know we were getting arrested to finding all of us a lawyer to help get our charges dropped. North Star even paid for all of us to have group therapy sessions, where we were free to process all the joy and fear that existed side by side that night.

We're not perfect, as North Star, in taking care of ourselves and each other. As we've doubled and tripled in size, and come through multiple years of upheaval and ongoing community actions of various types, we continue to work to find ways to hold each other in this for the long haul. We've tried all kinds of things from more casual hangouts to using outside facilitators, and are always open to new ideas. We don't take lightly that we have a lengthy fight ahead of us, and so we must take good care of everyone in the here and now. It's noteworthy in this regard that almost all the street medics, dispatchers, and other members of the collective are femme—literally over 95 percent. In a patriarchal society where many of us are also parents, adult children, nurses, and/or parts of chosen queer family, to care for ourselves while we care for our communities is a challenging yet radical act.

"I think being raised as a woman, I find myself doing things like I want to be the fixer or I want to support. I want to take

2. See "Cory Maria Dack, One of 11 Street Medics with North Star Health Collective Arrested during 'The People's Mandate' Protest on November 4, 2020," Unicorn Riot, https://vimeo.com/700701534.

things on. I want to meet your problems and create space for that in myself [even if] I don't even have it," remarks Em. "I have to separate that from my earnest desire to do good in the world. And I think North Star has been really helpful for that because I'm not taking anything on simply to do it. I feel good about this work and don't feel like I'm necessarily bringing gendered baggage."

"I feel like North Star does a great job of centering taking care of yourself too. That has been the vibe every time there's a protest," explains Parvaneh. "'You have a stomach ache? Don't medic that night.' I really respect and appreciate that because especially in other spaces that I've been in, it's just, 'Who can last out here the longest? I haven't eaten in four days. What about you? Don't you believe in the cause!' With North Star, it's chill."

## NORTH STAR TODAY, NORTH STAR TOMORROW

Minneapolis, the Twin Cities Metro, and the state of Minnesota are in a challenging moment right now. It's been nearly three years since the uprising in response to the lynching of George Floyd, followed by subsequent uprisings around the city, and almost two years since the culminating summer of frontline fights against the Line 3 pipeline. The amount of people being ground up while going through the legal system is staggering—somewhere in the thousands—not to mention the impact of trauma on those facing state repression and/or having been part of such battles. The work of trying to pick up the pieces and figure out what comes next, and how heavy that weight feels, is palpable. For all the broader attention that comes with the pitched battles and direct actions, there are a lot of attempts to do things differently that go unseen. There are struggles with resources (too many and too few), burnout, strategic and tactical differences of opinion, and an often exhausted crew of mutual aid folks working to keep up with the ongoing battles between unhoused people and the city's eviction campaigns.

This only scratches the surface of the work that we both try to care for and not destroy ourselves in doing. And it all comes with a lot of grief. It is one thing to say that we pushed to new levels when that precinct burned down; it's another to live here day-to-day with the police who continue to get more money and act with impunity. It's impressive to watch a community throw everything it has at the system (we even tried voting in a citywide referendum, one of the outcomes of the uprising, to "abolish" the police); it is also a hard reality to face that harm is still being caused and parents are still grieving their state-murdered children.

This is the moment we are trying to live into and build in right now—with our values in hand, no matter how that fight continues to play out. We do that in community relationships with other projects, collectives, and groups. We do that by taking time to dig into our own internal structure and makeup, aspiring to move into increasingly nonhierarchical structures balanced by listening to those with long experience in both North Star and our communities. As part of that, we've initiated an Anti-Racist Praxis Project within North Star.

North Star is built on a history and practice with defined ethics, and we train this and work to live it every day. We are not neutral. There's no test or ideological adherence required for entry, but most of us are anarchists, and we don't shy away from that word within our collective. Instead, we lean into what we are trying to build. We create a space where we use the words *anarchist* and *abolitionist*, underscoring that we're a largely femme and queer organization. Perhaps that is a key way in which we are deeply feminist: we are here to be in relationship with each other as we all grow together.

Within that, our roles change and shift. Some of us are over two decades in, and some of us have been part of North Star for three years or even three months. We recognize that organizing can be challenging and frequently inaccessible. How does a group that spans generations, and spans life experiences related to race, gender, culture, faith, and so much more, make space in a way that is open and welcoming? All we can do, as medics with North Star, is cup our hands around the flame, feel its warmth, and tend to that with care, and hope that what we strive to nurture continues to grow.

❊　❊　❊

Mags Beall is an organizer in the prefigurative anarchist tradition; she identifies as a queer femme who is a descendant of a mix of northern European (mostly Irish) settler colonizers. Over the past twenty-five years, she has engaged in local fights against ecological destruction and for animal liberation, (im)migrant solidarity and No More Deaths, antifascism, and housing. In 2015, she left the US West Coast, rejoining her blood family in Minnesota (unceded Dakota and Anishinaabeg territory), continuing with street medic and community health work. She continues to participate in mutual aid and radical movement work in the Twin Cities, working toward building a better world with better institutions, rooted in liberatory praxis. Mags would like to thank Cory, Cindy, countless friends, family, and collective mates, North Star, TLC, and especially, Alli, Betsy, Ed, Emma, Jayce, Kyle, Rach, and Sadie.

Cory Maria Dack is an Indigenous Latina from Ecuador and northern Minnesota. She recently led a full Source to Sea paddle of the Mississippi River to "decolonize thru-paddling" by increasing representation and uplifting the voices of women of color, immigrants, fat-bodied people, and members of the LGBTQ+ community. When not living in a canoe, she runs as a street medic with North Star Health Collective. Cory would like to thank her mentors at North Star for keeping her safe on the front lines, her friends and family for learning and growing with her, and her dad for always supporting her, even when some of the stuff she does scares him.

Mags and Cory would like to offer deep gratitude to the whole of North Star Health Collective. They also want to thank the collective friends and communities across the Twin Cities, Minnesota, and Turtle Island, especially all the fellow street medics they've learned so much from and who have offered them such support over the years, along with their collaborators in Relationships Evolving Possibilities and Voices for Radical Justice.

## STITCHING TOGETHER OTHER WORLDS

## /

CINDY BARUKH MILSTEIN

For those on the margins, making do with scraps is common sense.

I've no idea if that's what led me, as a preteen and teenager, to take bits of colorful fabric, cut them into triangles and trapezoids and other queered shapes, and stitch them into square patches. The idea was to someday craft enough that I could then sew them together into a patchwork quilt. I made neat, growing stacks of these patches, setting them aside in my closet. Over those years, I had more than enough for many quilts, many times over, but I never started, much less finished, even one.

In parallel with this solo activity, yet stretching back as far as I can remember, I was constantly dreaming up and bringing to life all sorts of otherworldly spaces, also pieced together from scraps, but collaboratively with others. To take just one early example, along with a crew of preteen pals, I self-organized our own theatrical adaptation of *Hansel and Gretel* using the basement of my house as our stage, and naturally felt it was a great idea to drag in hundreds of fallen tree branches that we scavenged outdoors to construct a full-on forest indoors. In our version, as I recall, we celebrated kids running away from insufferable situations and trying to live by caring for each other (via foraging and candy), with the witch as an accomplice—not villain. Yet the real magical transformation was that a dusty cellar filled with abandoned things could become a leafy wooded paradise overflowing with friends.

In hindsight, weaving beautiful social fabrics has been a contiguous thread running through my life. I realize now, though, why I never completed a quilt: one shouldn't have to do it alone; moreover, the insidiousness of how patriarchy socializes us all made me "feminize" and thus devalue my hand-sewn patches as any sort of contribution. It feels metaphorically accurate that I hid them away in a closet, making my own handiwork invisible. I didn't yet understand that every labor of love can be a small piece of something much bigger, wholly at cross-purposes with the current social order, when we intentionally and collectively suture those parts into a whole. We have all the material we need, right in our scrappy hands.

Take the implicitly rebellious history of quilting.

This "women's work" was, for centuries, not merely a necessity in terms of supplying households of modest means with blankets. Crucially, it allowed female and queer folks to create their own social, cultural, and political space in the form of what has come to be called "quilting bees." Here, those relegated to the so-called domestic sphere came together to collectivize their scraps and labor, literally and figuratively sewing communal comfort for each other, and in the process, making room for themselves in a world that typically shut them out. While stitching, they could exchange everything from recipes and home remedies, to their problems and fears, to news and gossip, or skills and other resources. They could tell each other stories of hardship or harm, and from there, lend each other protection or intervention; or swap stories of loss and grief, and offer emotional care; or spin tales of joy, dreams, and aspirations, likely fomenting all sorts of resistance to achieve their visions.

Frequently, these bees turned into community events, bringing what would otherwise be invisible efforts into the light of day, including via folks embroidering their own stories as images on quilts. That kind of radical comfort made its way, for instance, into the AIDS memorial quilt, an idea emerging from street demos following the 1978 assassination of gay San Francisco supervisor Harvey Milk and the resultant riots as a way to honor the dead and fight for the living during a "silence equals death" pandemic that killed off so many gay and gender-nonconforming people.

The point isn't that every quilt equals revolution. It's that we shouldn't minimize the potential of what can feel like small, individual patches of practices, whether on our own or with tiny circles of friends and neighbors. We shouldn't make invisible the kinds of liminal, messy-beautiful time-spaces we make for our crafting and scheming, whether they produce material embodiments as a result, and/or the essential immateriality of reciprocal comfort and care, aiding us to be coconspirators in mending this world. And when displayed together—like the AIDS quilt, which stretches for miles now and was toured at the start of another pandemic, COVID, which in turn sparked a wave of mutual aid and summer of uprising—we realize that we are indeed everything we need and want and desire. We ourselves sow possibilities, and ones that can get us through the coldest and darkest of days and nights.

So here's a small sampler—what's usually dismissed as ultimately forming a "crazy quilt," without design or intention, when viewed from the vantage point of heteronormativity, patriarchy, and other tools of violence that rip us to shreds. Yet through the lens of dignity, life, and freedom, it's the stuff of weaving a perfectly beautiful, anarcha-feminist pattern.[1]

# 1

The beloved project ended, badly. A monthlong anarchist camp—but so much more than that—that I'd thrown myself into for a decade's worth of summers. It split into two halves that could never again form a whole, if it ever did. More precisely, one half had to leave because the other half had, over the years, organized as if in a cloud-cuckoo-land, not wanting to venture past its own political dogmatism, internal power dynamics, and patriarchal behaviors (despite rhetoric to the contrary), or inability to deal with the reality of mundane logistics like paying the bills. Our half had brought vibrancy to this project, not only renewing it in many ways, but doing the lion's share of the self-organizing and communal care to make it happen. In the end, we became, to borrow from Ursula K. Le Guin, "the ones who walk[ed] away" from what had, for us, so often felt utopian, knowing that our departure also spelled the death of this longtime, remarkably transformative space for hundreds of other anarchists from around the world.

Similar to the conclusion of Le Guin's short story, we couldn't yet imagine what alternative universe we were journeying toward, though, mostly because our hearts were so heavy. "It is possible it does not exist," observes Le Guin.

---

1. This sampler is based solely on my own recollections, filtered through the mists of time, beginning with the first piece in the 1990s and early 2000s, and moving closer to the present from there. It does not mean to imply a seamless experience; like all feministic anarchist experiments, these have their share of flaws and heartbreaks. Still, it's crucial to recognize those time-spaces when we feel as if we're already inhabiting the kinds of social and organizational relations that we so desire and deserve.

"But they seem to know where they are going, the ones who walk away."

What we knew, as genderqueer friends and even chosen family, was that we had to process our loss together. We had to rest and regroup, play and rethink. And as part of that, on one sunny day, we circled up around a table outside a bakery in our tiny town, ourselves a tiny crew, to eat and brainstorm. What did we want to see emerge out of the ashes and lessons of the project we'd just left? Over the next year, five years, or even ten? And crucially, what did we want to promise each other about how to do the next project(s) differently so as to actually embody our ethics, especially around organizing as if social relations matter? Felt-tip markers transferred our musings onto big sheets of butcher-block paper, which quickly filled with seemingly unattainable strivings.

Soon after, serendipitously, some folks starting an anarchistic all-ages café and community hub asked if we wanted a small room on the second floor above them, along with access to hosting events in their space. Thus our all-volunteer, no-profit, collectively run Black Sheep Books was born, with both projects opening their doors on the same day. We eventually outgrew our spot and moved about a block away, into a storefront already painted black and red. And five years after our mutual grand opening, the café and Black Sheep ended, but well.

At some point during that time, us Black Sheepers looked over our now-rumpled list of dreams and were startled to realize that we'd achieved so much of what we wanted, materially, organizationally, and politically, plus ahead of "schedule." But what felt best was that we'd lived up to our promises, even when it was hard, or when each of us was going through tough times. Those promises were numerous, yet one jumps out in particular: entering into and exiting collective efforts with intentionality and empathy, and checking in every six months to be sure we all felt good about each other, what we were doing, and continuing to go forward together. This involved making good on our promises of, say, communal care and good communication, but importantly, it was grounded in our shared recognition that both the project and every one of us had to grow alongside each other, even if that meant consensually disassociating when Black Sheep wasn't nourishing for us, our communities, and/or our aims anymore.

So we had many an open and honest conversation in that last year, including through breakups, heartache, and depression, and knew that while Black Sheep could have forged ahead, it shouldn't. We ended while we still appreciated each other; we ended without being in debt, and in fact, seeded several other new anarchist projects in our town with the leftover funds; and we ended by each of us moving toward other horizons. It felt sad, yet in a way that could be integrated and didn't erase each other or the joy in what we'd created together. And it ended with an anarchistic marching band, going between the bookstore and café in a celebratory, musical "funeral" march for us and the community around us.

2

It was not a safe space. How could it (pretend to) be?

Not only was it smack-dab in the center of the intensive

war zone that was "gentrification," aka displacement and dispossession, in San Francisco. But our space was not immune from causing harm to ourselves and others. After all, every anarchist, no matter where they live, has been shaped and socialized in, and traumatized by, the violent social order.

Instead, from the first moment I pressed the doorbell on the grated-metal door, directly across the street from the chaos of the best and worst of humanity on the 16th Street BART Plaza, and looked through to see zines haphazardly tossed on a small shelf, then walked up the two interior flights of rundown stairs lined with militant posters from around the globe, to next enter into an enormous room decorated with banners and abuzz with activity—and vibrantly multipurposed as an infoshop, event, and organizing space as well as living room, kitchen, and set in the corner, bathrooms—it felt deeply like coming home. Then it became home. And now it may always be the closest thing to home for me, even though eviction stole it out of anarchist hands.

It felt homey precisely because everything feels unsafe in this world, and the Station 40 collective, through a rotating cast of twenty to twenty-four housemate-characters and countless guests, somehow squeezed into eight bedrooms and lots of nooks, held to this agreement: "We're not a safe space. But when shit happens, we promise to deal with it."

Because shit will and did happen. And dealing with that by not involving the cops and state, nor lashing out at each other, takes experimentation and dedication—including making mistakes—through the ins and outs of daily life. So while my housemates mostly prided themselves on being and going "hard," their demeanor extended to being rock-hard solid when it came to the "soft" practices of collective care and solidarity in ways I've rarely experienced before or after.

Station 40 was far from perfect, or easy, or always kind. It could feel like a war zone inside our doors, too, at times. "Shit" occurred routinely given that we were a hub for anarchism in the Bay Area at the time. Pretty much every intense thing that could happen, did happen. But I learned, time and again, that when the going gets excruciatingly tough, I wasn't alone, nor did I have to slip into being the lone caretaker. Moreover, "care work" was neither made invisible nor gendered but rather felt like the hearth, as it were, of our home—even if that care didn't look warm and fuzzy, such as false promises of "safe space." In fact, some of the housemates who showed me, personally, the most tender care and deep reciprocity had the crankiest, coldest, hardest shell (or so they fronted).

Yet those shells became shields of mutual self-defense and protection at a moment's notice when faced with threats to our house and/or potential perils to housemates, friends, and comrades. Our space—through which thousands of anarchists and like-minded folks passed, and that defied the typical face of anarchism given our eclectic and wide-ranging mix of races, cultures, genders, ages, and so much more that somehow meshed so well—almost invariably lived up in queer-feministic practice to the slogan "Be careful with each so we can be dangerous together."

That looked like, for example, knowing that our lengthy rectangular kitchen table—at the heart of Station 40—was open for any and all topics, including many that would have been off-limits or politically incorrect in most antiauthoritarian spaces. Over big meals or after 11:00 p.m. in particular, we spent many a night wrestling with dilemmas, in lively, provocative, and generative dialogues. Those raucous, no-holds-barred conversations helped us grow. Together, we felt comfortable scrutinizing and challenging various "safe" positions in the wider anarchist world—positions that other comrades frequently took up unthinkingly, for one, but also positions that ultimately put anarchists and others in further harm's way (for instance, via essentialized notions of identity that broke down our solidarities).

It looked, too, like us acting in concert, each playing their accomplished part without a conductor, such as when police suddenly raided our home during a big, crowded event. Everyone simultaneously leaped into action, taking on roles that fit their skill sets. That meant that we had everything we needed, within minutes, to lockdown our space, mobilize lawyers and community to show up outside, and spirit away what or who needed special protection while deciding on our strategy, yet equally, to calm our many guests and offer emotional support as needed.

Or it looked like us collectively fighting outbreaks of bedbugs, eradicating the infestations by relying on our own research and self-organization, being transparent with the wider community and at times responsibly shutting down our space to visitors, and aiding each other with the many tedious tasks necessary to ensure success. It meant trying to turn this tragedy into humor as well, from dubbing it our "social war" to jokingly imagining our neighbors all setting their bedbug-infested mattresses alight at intersections for a street party against evictions to scare off the invasive tech bros driving rents sky high.

Or it looked like intimate caretaking in the most unsafe of situations for an individual, such as our whole collective holding empathetic space for a housemate actively contemplating suicide over a twenty-four-hour period and finding them the consensual resources they needed to decide to live.

Shit happened. And together, we got through it as safely as possible.

### 3

Maybe it was the open, multilevel, hundred-plus-year-old barn that sparked our "cultivating care" framework. After all, anyone driving by it on the wooded road, friend or foe, could see right into the charmingly ramshackle structure, making this now-longtime radical space feel equal parts beautiful and vulnerable. It was clearly a magical location for our anarchist summer school. But the magic wasn't simply "there," like this barn, built decades ago by unknown others. As an organizing collective, we had to continually tend to the floorboards and support beams, literally and figuratively, to conjure it up. And that ongoing "repair work" had to be something that everyone who participated in the camp for three summers proactively engaged in side by side.

How, though, could we encourage everyone to be tinkerers, and with what tool kits? There were so many devices we wanted to pack into the programming—history, strategic thinking, hands-on skills related to direct action, play, and more. Way too much for an eight-day camp. Yet perhaps the most crucial tool turned out to be something that is not usually ready to hand in most anarchist spaces: being vulnerable with each other, and doing so as the foundation for everything else.

From the opening circle on, held in the embrace of the ancient barnwood that had once been a canopy of trees for other ecosystems, we welcomed and modeled the painstaking yet joyful work of everyone striving to be the person they aspire to be, sharing the fullness of themselves and their gifts. We took up what might seem like antiquated tools—such as opening up our hearts and minds to each other, challenging ourselves to grow in generative ways including by leaning into discomfort, and remembering that anarchism and life are messy-beautiful processes—so as to see and get to know each other as multidimensional, messy-beautiful people. We emphasized that community isn't a prefab, static entity; it's something we all directly and dynamically cultivate together. So we invited everyone, for the duration of camp, to experiment wholeheartedly, tenderly, and in ways we usually only dream about with "caring for each other like we're already in a new, do-it-ourselves world."

That's how the magic appeared. Which is another way of saying that otherworldly social relations emerged.

On that ground, we experienced all sorts of otherworldly conversations, dances, campfires, rituals, and silliness, otherworldly learning, adventuring, grieving, and creating, otherworldly good troublemaking and inspiration. And when we stumbled into difficult territory over the course of those three summers in that barn, we chose otherworldly ways of journeying through it. We chose empathy and trust. We chose love.[2]

So during our last, prepandemic summer when one

---

2. I'm borrowing loosely from the title of Kai Cheng Thom's *I Hope We Choose Love: A Trans Girl's Notes from the End of the World* (Vancouver: Arsenal Pulp Press, 2019).

participant ignored many people's boundaries—from emotional to logistical, material to physical—and kept violating consent, we chose to see everyone—all of us—as perfectly imperfect people always capable of transformation. We chose to strive to not merely do no further harm but rather aid each other in breaking patterns that arise from and/or cause trauma in ourselves and others. And even though we had, in the end, to ask that person to leave camp, we didn't dehumanize them or leave them out of these aspirations. Instead, we let love guide us.

The ins and outs of how we did this aren't reducible to a how-to list, in the same way that love can't and shouldn't be quantified. That's almost certainly why this "accountability process" worked better than the vast majority of them. It wasn't a formulaic process; instead, it was embedded in bonds of love, expansively understood and intentionally nurtured by everyone's willingness to open up to and with each other. As such, we didn't begin or end by broadcasting rumor or drama to the whole camp. We didn't cancel anyone or make anyone disposable. We didn't think or act through binaries of good/ bad, nor a carceral or punishment logic.

We listened. We believed. We held space for everyone's life stories, including the person who was pushing boundaries, and how people's past experiences shaped their present behaviors, feelings, and reactions. We held space, too, for how violations of consent can bring up a lot for everyone, whether receiver, giver, or eyewitness to the harm. We brought curiosity to how those stories and experiences can butt up against each other, intentionally or not, and how much this world that we so long to change has such power to turn us into people we don't want to be or can't see we've become.

Almost organically, like gently tossing a pebble into a mirrorlike pond and letting interdependent circles ripple outward, we threw ourselves compassionately and self-reflectively into the fabric of our social relations, which we'd been cultivating before and during camp, and let circles of mutualistic care ripple outward. Those circles let us each take on what we felt we could, and what we felt we could contribute, and equally at times, encircled us when we couldn't take on various tasks, or even more profoundly, helped us see when we couldn't or shouldn't take on various tasks. Those circles embraced everyone in differential yet interdependent ways, during and well beyond camp, including the person who seemingly couldn't maintain boundaries. And those circles—the ones we ourselves had built—saw us all as deserving of dignity, solidarity, and love, even if we need to not share space sometimes.

## 4

Richard Spencer's cross-country speaking tour at US colleges was put to a screeching halt by thousands of "little" acts of antifascist care.

Of course, what the headlines will tell you is quite different: "Violence Erupts on MSU Campus as Richard Spencer Speaks"; "Fights Break out at Michigan State [University] as Protesters, White Supremacists Converge for Richard Spencer Speech." And alas, some of the more bro-ey antifascists among us who contributed to this wildly successful deplatforming effort would largely agree, pointing to the fighting—the physical community self-defense—as what did the trick on

March 5, 2018. Not that throwing punches at a neo-Nazi, antisemitic conspiracy theorist, and white supremacist such as Spencer is bad or wrong; often it's strategically wise and tactically necessary. Fascism tends not to listen to "reasoned" arguments, contrary to what liberals like to believe.

But sometimes liberals, including progressive and social democratic ones, can be moved by compelling arguments to actively and consensually take direct action against fascism. And so when we heard Spencer's tour was slated to come to East Lansing, and anarchist(ic) folks knew that if we hoped to squash his mobilization, we needed large numbers of people—far beyond our confederation of anarchist groups in a half-dozen Michigan cities—we spent months making those arguments in a form that might not be recognizable as such. We asserted, in deeds not words, solidarity and care.

That wasn't without some contention with our own anarchist circles. Strains of machismo maintained that "care" wasn't radical. That attitude, in turn, meant that some patriarchal behaviors crept in, elevating "defense" and those who prioritized it, while at times denying "solidarity" to those of us focusing on communal care (though never doing so on the streets thankfully). Remarkably, however, we all understood the big picture—smashing fascism—and the necessity of outreach to build momentum and, on the big day, numbers. So ultimately, for and through this antifascist win, we all took care (double meaning intended!) to make it work, before, during, and after #StopSpencer.

This manifested in so many ways, it would be impossible to capture them all, and such tender direct actions of care are better lived than described. But a few examples should provide an idea.

*Before*: The collective I was part of, in the town with the most amount of organizing toward March 5, joined in a coalition among a wide range of political tendencies, with the majority of folks falling somewhere on the liberal spectrum, new to activism, never mind antifascism. Many had never been to a demonstration, or at least not one where the risk of heavily armed cops and fascists was so palpable. Our collective already had the trust of most activists in our town due to how we'd consistently shown up, and as the most imaginative, savvy, and welcoming of mischief makers. We put that trust to work, with patience and humility, first listening to why most people in the coalition were so hesitant to actually be present in person to #StopSpencer; second, really hearing and believing them, with empathy not annoyance; and finally, offering weeks of mentorship. Because when we listened, it came down to two reasons: not so much their liberal or social democratic sensibilities, as we'd thought, but fear and lack of experience. Through trainings, one-on-one conversations, and myriad other support, we gave them the knowledge, skills, and wisdom to feel empowered to be there on March 5, on whatever terms and by taking up whatever roles felt most consensual to them. The result was not simply that our city brought out the most people, and in affinity crews, but also that those folks felt as comfortable and prepared as one can when facing off with cops and fascists.

*During*: As we'd taught other affinity groups to do, my collective had spent hours ahead of time talking honestly about our fears and preferred levels of engagement at #StopSpencer. Based on that, we'd created layers of a buddy system, off-site meeting point, secure communication, jail support forms, and backup plans, among other things, plus we had agreed to arrive and leave together. And we did that over a fun evening of banner making and food in the warmth of a collective member's house, further nourishing our friendships and the deep culture of care among us. On the "battlefield" (in this case, a cornfield behind what's known as Moo U) that March 5, our bonds meant that we could simply look each other in the eye and know what needed to dynamically shift or who needed extra solidarity. All the care work put into building the #StopSpencer coalition and other statewide social relationships among organizers, though, meant that many of us—beyond our own affinity crews—could do the same. Time and again, through eye contact or body language, people aided others in calming down or stepping back when needed, or crews felt braver than anticipated and moved closer to the front line with the complementary support of other affinity groups. In the heat and intensity of this real battle, communal defense was inseparable from communal care.

*After*: It wasn't planned, but in the week after #StopSpencer, we not only celebrated what was a victory on multiple levels—Spencer canceled his tour, some prominent fascist groups unraveled, no one was shot or killed by cops or white supremacists (a real worry), and we forged loads of new mutualistic infrastructure and projects, to name some. We also dived gratefully into one debrief after another, large and small, in public spaces and private ones. For even though we won, the tension and trauma of being so close to heavily armed cops and fascists still brought up big feelings. Three things stuck out during our debriefs. People were deeply committed to this form of aftercare, showing up as their whole, vulnerable selves with and for each other. Most of those who weren't or hadn't previously been anarchists before #StopSpencer credited us anarchists with supplying the care and solidarity they needed to find their own strength, allowing them to go further than they ever thought they could. And crucially, processing together works wonders.

Care works, including in the fight to hinder fascism.

**5**

There were so many times during #DefendJ20 when it felt like the state was sitting back, laughing at us, watching codefendants and their supporters tear each other apart. I knew it was the intense emotional strain of some two hundred people facing the possibility of seventy-five years behind bars after being mass arrested during #Disrupt20 at Trump's 2017 inauguration that caused the internal fractures, acrimony, and even downright nastiness as the weeks turned into months of us trying to sustain our DIY solidarity infrastructure. It's not that J20 codefendants weren't supported with a tremendous amount of love and solidarity—legal, material, and immaterial. But on the regular, there wasn't a feministic commitment to gently, skillfully, and carefully intervening at the first sign that the statist stress was being misplaced onto our own dynamics.

To this day, I'm proud that a core of us supporters—"coincidentally," a majority of which were queer and/or female—stuck it out, even if the end was bittersweet: collective defense mostly held and the charges were dropped, thank goodness, but unprocessed trauma and antagonisms within ex-J20 circles lingered on.

State repression is good for that: first creating immense fear among those targeted, then dragging out the costly (to us) proceedings, and then waiting for the fear itself to do the work of destroying or at least severely harming us.

But not always. Maybe we've learned, including from our mistakes.

Take #StopCopCity in so-called Atlanta. For all the many imaginative "diversity of tactics" that have so marked this inspiring movement over the past couple of years, perhaps the most overlooked is its self-generated "culture of care," which seems to be almost a given, especially within the solidarity efforts. The more that the cops, courts, and governments have ramped up serious, albeit absurd, charges against forest defenders, and particularly after the statist assassination of Tortuguita on January 18, 2023, mourning ceremonies and communal rituals, in-person care clinics, mutual aid therapy and peer-to-peer emotional support, medicinal herbs, and various other healing arts have only multiplied. Like everything else in this struggle to #DefendTheWeelauneeForest, all of this care is autonomously self-organized and offered with a generosity of spirit as well as prefigurative sensibility.

Those bigger, more visible direct actions of care are touching, of course, and go a long way to explaining why #Stop-CopCity has not only captured so many hearts and minds but also been so relatively long-lived, growing to embrace people from many different walks of life. What's felt so transformative, though, are the innumerable smaller, everyday direct actions of care that seem hardly worth remarking on or even taking note of—not out of lack of appreciation, but because they've coalesced into a shared culture of communal care that we're now so deeply embedded in, it's like the air we breathe within the solidarity efforts. Or more precisely, it's like a warm hug when things feel stressful—or for that matter, joyful too, or indeed when things feel all sorts of ways because of the ravages of state repression.

To take a few "breaths" as examples:

When a large Signal thread full of supporters started filling up with gratuitously mean-spirited texts related to some genuine conundrum we were grappling with, one person matter-of-factly observed that the state has a long history of employing counterintelligence tactics against us. They noted that we can and should engage in disagreements over tough issues, but in ways that don't play into the state's divide-and-conquer schemes. Not only did this single, succinct text serve to de-escalate; it almost immediately reinstalled a sense of shared purpose.

When in order to "do our job" (voluntarily of course) as jail support folks, we had to watch hours of court hearings on live YouTube feeds, with our comrades, movement, and politics being painted by the red-baiting prosecutor as "terrorist," two therapists held a virtual "processing space" afterward. Not only did this single, humble session gift us with something we didn't even think we needed, but once we began talking/crying, we clearly did; it fast reaffirmed that we, too, as solidarity "workers" were seen and appreciated.

When a family member of a current codefendant was falling apart from worry about their beloved, a family member of a now ex-codefendant from the J20 days spoke with them. Not only did this single, modest phone call hopefully go a little way to supplying the kind of empathy and understanding that only comes from a shared, unique experience; it repaid forward something that this J20 family member had constructively critiqued as wanting for themselves and not getting back then—that is, support for the impacts on the codefendants' kin.

Indeed, when folks see that someone in our solidarity circles, no matter their role, is struggling—such as because of a fresh loss, mental health challenge, or overwhelm and exhaustion—it's almost commonplace to simply reach out to them, one on one—if at a distance, by sending a loving voice message, say; if nearby, by putting a consensual arm around their shoulder and encouraging them to breathe. Not only do these single, simple gestures aid in deactivating some of the worst edges of, for instance, grief or anxiety; they almost instantly reinstill feelings of not being alone, or conversely, being interconnected.

Or when rumors begin to fly, there seems to always be someone offering a calm reminder that we can deal with any solid information that arises—we have everything we need among us to handle what gets thrown at us—but that rumors only whip up fear and panic, and can lead to harming other supporters/codefendants, breaking trust, and/or making hasty, bad decisions. Or someone will serenely volunteer to look into the rumor and follow up with facts. Not only do these single, levelheaded responses ease the added emotional turmoil that rumors catalyze; they quickly reinscribe the knowledge that a lot of folks, with a ton of skills and savvy, are engaging in joint defense, whether legally or ethically.

Each of these minor interactions—most taking only a few minutes—have to date, time and time again, not only held our solidarity in place. They seem to be mitigating unnecessary suffering—the kind we too often inflict on each other when the boot of repression presses down on us, rather than directing our hostilities at the correct target, the state—while accentuating the quality of care we see as simply the culture of everyday anarchism.

When the charges are hopefully all dropped, it's possible to already imagine this culture carrying forward, as second nature, into the next battle.

**6**

The two most joyous anarchist gatherings I've experienced since the pandemic began both made the most amount of room for grief. And I wasn't alone in that assessment.

That might sound paradoxical. How can sorrow and joy commingle? How can we find the greatest sense of a harmonious whole by publicly curating space for both anguish and delight?

For most of human history, people practiced an abundance of intricate, culturally embedded communal rituals and sacred spaces to not only get them through every transition, good and bad, but also make sense of those shifts. Such ceremonies, from festivals to funerals, were inseparable parts of a healthy ecosystem. They (re)generated, sustained, and affirmed life and its cycles, giving them dignity and meaning. They let people immerse themselves in the entire spectrum of human emotions, which in actuality don't fit neatly into experiences but instead are bound up in the highs and lows of them all.

Alas, among the many wisdoms lost when our elaborate rituals were stolen over the centuries by the powers-that-be, whether by assimilation or annihilation, was this: rituals, which bring out all the pieces of ourselves, are essential as the reparative and restorative glue of fully living.

Contemporary anarchism has, to its detriment, followed too obediently in the footsteps of the hegemonic death-denying culture we've been boxed into, largely abandoning rituals, most especially ones related to grief, and leaving our losses and feelings around them largely unprocessed. When unprocessed, feelings don't just go away. They build up until they explode—whether inside ourselves and/or at each other.

Those "explosions" have been keenly palpable since the onset of COVID-19. The numbers of suicides, road-rage accidents, overdoses, and the like have skyrocketed, even as the dominant culture—so adept at producing mass death—further isolated folks from each other and urged a return to "normal." Anarchists, too, yearned to go back to our normal, such as bookfairs and social centers, uprisings and frontline camps, but vastly underestimated how much the collective trauma had touched us, and thus did little to deeply think through, much less implement, what needed to shift in our own convergences. And with little to no ritualistic mechanisms to fall back on to journey through our own layers of loss and grief together, too many anarchists blew up at each other, destroyed their own beloved projects, and further dissociated from their own sorrow as well as joy.

This attitude of ignoring grief at our own peril really hit home for me, personally and painfully, some eleven years ago, when I needed to caretake my simultaneously dying parents for about thirteen months. I thought I had a big, solid anarchist community, but it disappeared almost overnight. I was met instead with, "Come back when you're done," as if death and mourning were somehow outside our circles and friendships, and as if we could or should ever be "done" with grief, which is another name for what we love. That's why I threw myself into "rebellious mourning," in words and deeds, soon afterward.[3] Because too much of what we love—the majority, I'd argue—is unnecessarily taken from us by this death cult of a social order. When we explicitly mourn our losses, as part and parcel of everything else we self-organize, we're extra clear-eyed about what and for whom we're fighting, from the living to our ancestors; we proactively mend ourselves and this world; and we keep love and life at the heart of all we do. Moreover, we're far better able to stick side by side with each other, tightening our interrelationships so as to get through the most excruciating of times.

Still, I often felt too alone in that task while wandering around doing hundreds of grief circles, and felt "crazy" seeing how much damage was wrought by us not doing the collective work of grief. Yet I was wrong. I wasn't completely alone; other anarchists had also felt called toward this task. And to wind my way back to those two, most joyous of anarchist events—Another Carolina Anarchist Bookfair (ACAB) and the Montreal Anarchist Bookfair—those isolated labors had now coalesced into shared efforts. Making space for grief was as integral a component as, say, tabling, food, and parties, thanks especially to feministic anarchists on both collectives.

At ACAB, held in Asheville in August 2023, the organizing

---

3. Cindy Milstein, ed., *Rebellious Mourning: The Collective Work of Grief* (Oakland, CA: AK Press, 2017).

collective had intentionally scheduled not just one but instead three workshops related to dying, death, and mourning, with my grief circle kicking off the bookfair to set the tone. A regional collective that includes anarchist gravediggers and casket makers was invited to craft a custom altar, which sat outside the front door of Firestorm Books, one of the main venues for the entire weekend. And given that ACAB's first day fell on the sixth anniversary of Charlottesville, a friend from nearby Durham, NC, brought an enormous banner made around that time that read, "We struggle in memory of all we've lost to white supremacy and fascism." The banner was painted soon after Heather Heyer was murdered, and so many others were deeply injured and forever scarred, by fascists during the Unite the Right in August 2017. It was originally hung from the ten-foot-high stone base of the first Confederate monument that folks tore down in North Carolina, and later, on the one-year anniversary of that monument falling, it was hung up again—this time as part of an altar with names and flowers and candles around it, and folks read the names of people killed by the police in Durham. The banner took pride of place at ACAB, draped from Firestorm's rafters as background for workshops—including "Herbs for the Cycles of Grief" and "Radical Death Care"—and still hangs there to this day, honoring our dead on a daily basis alongside all the standard pleasures of an anarcha-feminist, queer+trans bookstore.

To wander back a bit further in time to February 2023, when those of us on the Montreal Anarchist Bookfair collective were in planning mode, I ran across three queer and/or female anarchists who all wanted to do a grief space. It was not only the dead of winter in a cold city but we were also grappling with recent heavy losses and didn't feel up to going out, so we met on Jitsi, having never met each other before. Over the course of an hour, the body language went from the equivalent of wrapped in a blanket on a couch, slumped over, barely able to look up or participate, to eye contact, enthusiasm, and warmth, leaning toward each other. We went from hardly motivated to being able to brainstorm a long list of great ideas. In between, without really intending to, we'd basically held a grief space for ourselves "simply" by talking about what we wanted and needed in one for others. We came with sorrow, and found joy too, and it was as if we'd known each other a long time.

Fast-forward to the bookfair in May 2023, and our little collective set up the biggest, most beautiful grief space I've yet to have the honor of helping to create—and not only that, but it was a sheer pleasure to organize from start to finish. Collectively, we had everything we needed to implement all of our many ideas; we allowed for a plurality of grief modalities and ways of approaching mourning; and when the bookfair was wrapping up, we sat in a circle inside our space to talk about our feelings, what went well, and what we wanted to do better next year—because we already envisioned a future together.

The space itself, outdoors near the main entrance to this gigantic bookfair for the entirety of the weekend, was composed of two pop-up tents with flowing DIY walls of fabrics and gorgeous hand-painted "grief" banners on the outside, along with a table of free anarchistic zines related to suicide, dying, death, and mourning. Inside, we constructed a "floor" of blankets and soft cushions, asked folks to take off their shoes when entering, and artfully laid out all sorts of participatory materials for mourning, from an altar to musical instruments and art supplies. We offered two programmed times—one focusing on somatics, and the other on talk—but for most of the time, we let folks engage with the space as they needed, with one of us on hand to hold space as desired. Mostly, we witnessed how people brought all of their senses to bear on the space—from sights and sounds, to smells and touch—and all of their emotions—ranging from tears and rage to laughter and love.

What struck me at both bookfairs was how many people—folks I didn't know, and who didn't know me, and had no idea I was part of any of the grief spaces—eagerly wanted to share their joy with me at being there. They went on and on about how friendly we anarchists were being toward each other, across all tendencies, offering genuine warmth, playfulness, and openness. They remarked on how refreshed, reconnected, and hopeful they felt thanks to these gatherings, in contrast to the past three years of despair and loss of faith.

I could relay story after story, but one suffices as illustration.

At a magical afterparty held at an enormous community space won through two decades of struggle, one particularly exuberant young person was gushing to me about their day at the Montreal Anarchist Bookfair. "I feel such joy, I can hardly express it," they said, beaming from ear to ear. I asked them to give me an example and suddenly their face turned somber. They spoke of having to fend off fascists in their small town with their small collective for the past three years, amid all the pandemic isolation, and how bleak everything felt before this weekend. "I wasn't sure I was up for a huge event and lots of socializing. Then I saw that grief space. I didn't go in. It was enough to see it and have it there. To have my grief made visible and acknowledged. That felt so genuine, which felt so joyful. It opened me up to joy again." A broad smile returned to their face. "Why do we hide grief? It has such power to bring and keep us together."

❋  ❋  ❋

Ten years ago, in the blink of an eye between my dad dying and my mom soon to follow, I was tasked with cleaning out their home of many decades as part of caring for them through sickness and death. The easiest solution, and most intuitively anarchistic one, was to do a make-an-offer "yard sale" right in the house itself. Yet in the down-and-out economy of Michigan, it quickly became apparent I needed to turn it into a really, really free market. Over the course of a week, hundreds of folks dug through the whole house from attic to the basement—the one I'd remade into a theater/forest so long ago—and took what they wanted. In the process, people told me their hard-luck stories, and I listened; then they wanted to hear about my losses, and they listened.

They also joyfully shared their finds with me, from a teenager who eagerly snagged the same typewriter I'd used as a teen, saying they wanted to be a writer, to the people without health insurance who'd discovered leftover medical supplies from my parents' illnesses that they themselves greatly needed, to the person who carted off what to me looked like sheer garbage, saving me the trouble.

Toward the end, one person lugged a dilapidated, musty cardboard box up from the cellar and plopped it in front of me. A huge grin spread across their face as they opened the box to reveal hundreds of fabric patches, a bit faded, but still bringing together geometries of purple and turquoise, pink and green, red and black, into pleasing designs. "Wow, I love these! Can I take them home?" they exclaimed. "Maybe I can invite a bunch of my friends over for a potluck and together we can all make a quilt!"

❖ ❖ ❖

Cindy Barukh Milstein still doesn't quilt. Or maybe they do, in different ways.

# ILLUSTRATING
# ANARCHA-FEMINISM

FIND EACH OTHER

DEFEND EACH OTHER

FREEDOM · AUTONOMY · JOY

# ADDY

I felt inspired to draw this because I wanted to express that we're out here. In my experience, it can feel lonely trying to find other people. Yet I have found and we will find people who understand how deeply we need each other, who want to grow together, to acknowledge that we're going to make mistakes and are capable of harming others, but will support each other with love, care, accountability, and tenderness to unlearn ways of thinking that are hurting us, and create safe, loving, anarchistic relationships and joyful realities. I created this illustration to print as a sticker and paste around my city, although I'm still looking for a printer that uses vegan materials, is worker owned, and has as little ecological footprint as possible.

My drawings are representations of my dreams of building another world as well as protesting against hierarchy (patriarchy included), speciesism, adult supremacy (that's why most of my characters look young), binaries, and the academy. They are about tenderness and vulnerability, about allowing us to feel rage and sadness, let our emotions bring us closer, and take care of and defend each other.

❊ ❊ ❊

Addy (she/her) loves drawing, taking naps, eating plants, looking at the world, making mistakes, and learning to live in community. You can find more of her drawings on Instagram @addy_rivera.

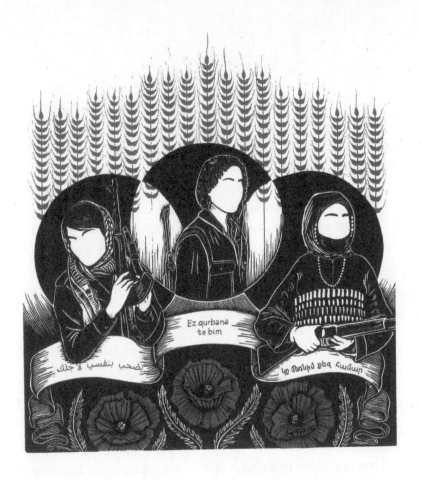

# ALI CAT

This print, *Our Promise*, celebrates a solidarity that exists beyond borders, spotlighting fights around the globe for land, dignity, and self-determination. Specifically, it honors women who have sacrificed their lives in these struggles. The figures portrayed here represent 1960s' Palestinian (*left*), 2000s' Kurdish (*center*), and 1880s' Armenian (*right*) resistance. The three individuals are accompanied by the phrase "I would die for you," in Arabic, Kurdish, and Armenian (*left to right*)—a powerful expression of affection used in Southwest Asia and North Africa (SWANA) regions.

Our promise: we will remember and uplift all of those women who battle tyranny and fascism. Our promise: we will never forget you, Shireen Abu Akleh, Jina Amini, and Anush Apetyan, who all lost their lives in 2022 due to occupation, domination, and colonization. Our promise: we will honor those who came before us and support those striving for liberation today.

❊ ❊ ❊

Ali Cat produces her work under the name Entangled Roots Press. Her relief, screen, and letterpress prints span themes from the tenderness of cultural reclamation to the beauty of people's movements. Ali's prints pull from ancestral herstories and push toward liberatory futures, entangling lessons from gardens, symbols in coffee cups, and woven threads from Armenia and Argentina to the printed page. You can find Ali's art on Instagram @entangledrootspress.

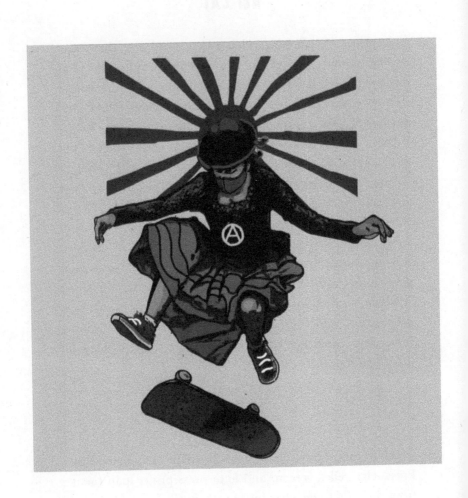

# AMAN

This image was inspired by a group of young skaters of Bolivian Indigenous origin, ImillaSkate (*imilla* means "young" in Aymara and Quechua). Through skateboarding, they give new meaning to the role of Latina women without losing sight of our traditions, culture, and resistance, nor the insurgency of our people against bloody colonialism.

My artwork portraying feminism reflects my own trajectory, treaded for years alongside rural, Indigenous, quilomba, riverside, and landless women, who also stand side by side with those women fighting in big cities for the fall of patriarchy, capital, and the state. I've learned that an Indigenous Kaiowá compañera's struggle is the same as that of a compañera in Rojava, and that a woman without land defends the caboclo seed like a Zapatista woman does too. I create art linked to community self-defense movements from Latin America to Africa and Asia as well as struggles for land and water, honoring the experiences, barricades, and memories of rebellion in Abya Yala, the original and ancestral name for the Western Hemisphere.

❧ ❧ ❧

I am Aman, which in Guajajara means "rain." I received this name because I'm part of a group of popular communicators and educators from traditional communities seeking to create strategies to defend our fields, rivers, and forests. You can find more of my art in the street, or on social networks like Twitter, Facebook, and Instagram @amanposters, or https://linktr.ee/AmanPosters.

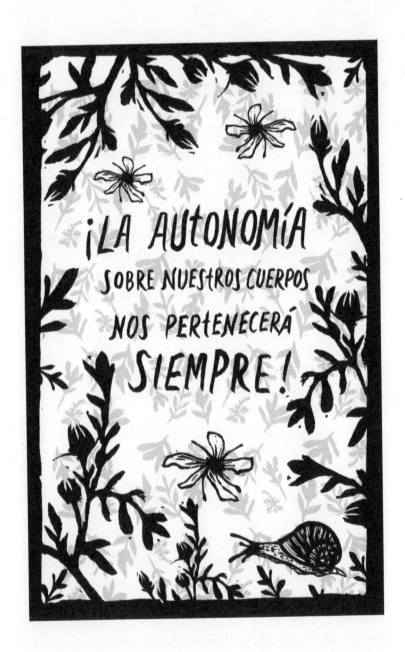

# ANDREA NARNO

"*Autonomía*, autonomy, our bodies will always belong to us," repeated as a chant in my mind while I created this image. With *Roe v. Wade*'s overturn and the attacks on gender-affirming care, the capacity and right to decide for oneself becomes disputed, preventing us from moving freely and reaching the horizons we dream of. In this harsh landscape, uplifting self-determination is an everyday task.

I hold tight to the love in the collective efforts to care for one another, to show up and share the bounties of our gardens. I look back into herbalism and ancestry practices as our paths toward healing. In this print, I dream of and portray an endless cascade of possibilities and autonomy for us all.

❊  ❊  ❊

Andrea Narno, a Mexican queer printmaker living in New Orleans, Louisiana, believes in art as a tool for transformation during these uncertain times. Their work centers around the symbolism of plants to express thoughts, feelings, and ideas as well as examine topics like migration, absence, and grief. Andrea is a member of Justseeds' Artist Cooperative. Alongside artist V Adams, they run Birds of Paradise Press, a project exploring distance, longing, and the connections we have to place through our relationships with plants. You can find them on Instagram @graficanarno.

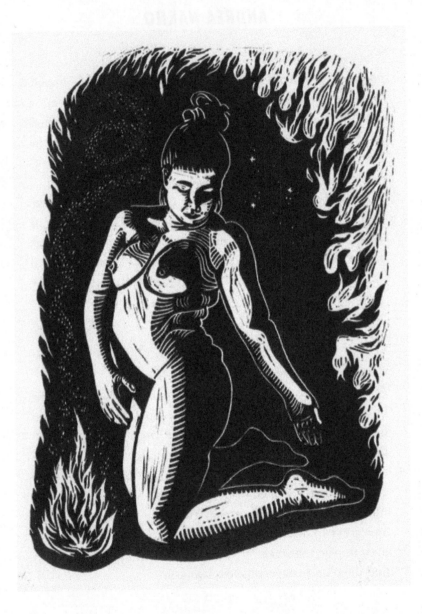

# ANOUK KUONA

The fire that we feed with our rage, our voices, and solidarity is the same flame that keeps me warm in cold nights. This linocut, *Chispas – Sparks – Funken*, summons this feeling. Every time we stick together, defending and holding each other, this roaring flame only grows stronger. It's the same fire that keeps us alive as activists; our connection is fueled by warmth, care, and tenderness.

I live in a small, conservative town, where it's hard work to sustain our feminist network. It's often exhausting to build structures for the first time here, and sometimes it's easy to feel alone, isolated from the larger, more established movements in the bigger cities. I create images in an attempt to overcome the separation between local and international struggles. I strive to offer a common language of love and rage as a reminder that although we may be few in my town, we're far from alone.

❀　❀　❀

Anouk Kuona is a self-taught printmaker and illustrator, born, raised, and currently living in southern Germany close to Landshut. She learned about printmaking while living in Mexico for several years and now makes art from her small workshop on a collectively owned farm in the countryside. Her prints frequently talk about feminist and anarchist topics. You can find her work on Instagram @anouk.kuona.prints.

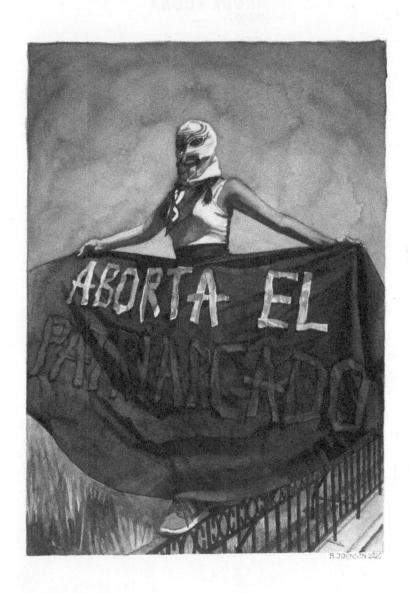

# BREE BUSK

International Women's Day on March 8 (8M) has become sacred for those of us still riding the wave of this ongoing feminist uprising. Although we mobilize all year round, 8M is when we can celebrate the size and strength of our movement, and flood the streets with our liberated bodies. Together, we can wear as much or as little as we want; we can paint our politics on our skin or embroider our slogans into our costumes. On 8M, you can hear our voices, but our bodies talk too. This watercolor captures a fragment of the spirit that animates us: a smiling young feminist balances on a fence while proudly displaying her hand-stitched violet-colored skirt, which reads, "Abort the patriarchy!"

My work, like my politics, is intensely personal, as my paintings are often intimate portraits of my friends and compañeras in the context of our feminist activism. Yet my work also features slogans, symbols, and performances that reference both local campaigns and global struggles against all forms of domination. This dichotomy speaks directly to my anarchist-feminist ethic since my art is an exploration of the interplay between the politics of everyday life and our collective ambitions for a utopian future.

❊  ❊  ❊

Bree Busk is an anarchist, artist, and writer based in Santiago, Chile, where she participates in the Coordinadora Feminista 8M. Bree's writing can be found at https://linktr.ee/breeatlast, and her art on Instagram @breeatlast.

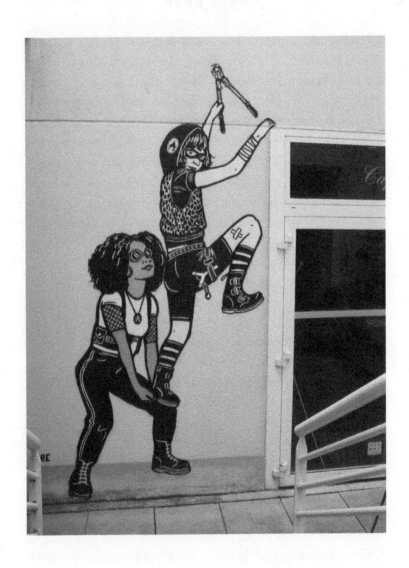

# ERRE

A year ago, I was traveling around different cities, as always with the aim of putting my graphic work in the streets, and learning and creating alongside like-minded projects. In Paris, I was invited to paint a mural on the exterior wall of a self-managed social center. This image was inspired by my experience of being able to journey widely only because of the mutual aid and solidarity of many friends, old and new. It was also inspired by the social center, which offers social support as well as cultural and education activities all based on solidarity, exchange, and sharing. As I drew the image, lyrics from the punk band Sham 69 came to mind: "If the kids are united, then we'll never be divided."

My work emerges from personal things mixed with social problems, using art against oppression, hierarchy, and inequality so as to invite people to unlearn practices and lose their fears, and instead speak up with complete autonomy.

❖ ❖ ❖

Erre, a street artist and illustrator, has been creating graphics and interventions in public spaces through a stencil technique for more than a decade in various cities around the world. Erre's work focuses on the energy and power of women. Each piece seeks to challenge patriarchy and authority, encouraging and inviting women to rise up, scream, act, and explode. You can find Erre's art on Instagram @erre.erre and at www.erre.com.co.

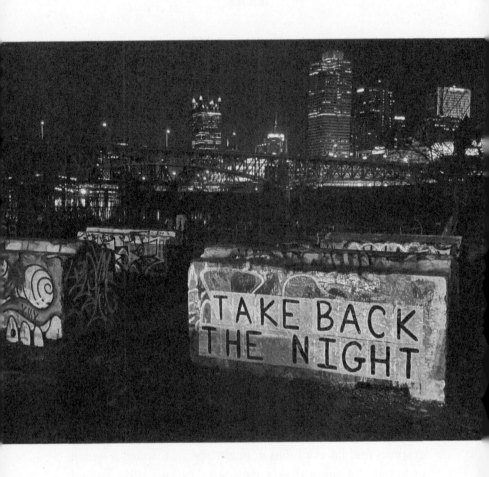

# FEMINIST COLLAGES PGH

The slogan "Take Back the Night" came from a 1970s' movement against all forms of sexual violence. In this case, it's tied directly to Dee, one of our collective members, whose mother was an active volunteer with Pittsburgh Action against Rape in the 1980s and 1990s, and went on Take Back the Night marches. For Dee, the slogan means "still here and still taking back the night," and the paste honors their mom, who died in 2018.

Feminist Collages PGH emerged after one of our collective members spent time in New York City in 2022 and saw wheat-pasted feminist phrases there. After doing online research, we found out that people were putting up similar street art around the world and began doing the same in Pittsburgh in January 2023. The wheat pastes—relatively easy and affordable to make by copying individual letters onto white paper—are a direct action to make our voices recognized and heard, because as cis and trans women, we're so often told to be quiet. The history of feminist collages started with a call to end femicide in particular—a topic that's rarely talked about and definitely never mentioned in Pittsburgh. Our goal is to raise awareness of things not typically spoken about in public and help bring an end to the violence of patriarchy.

❁ ❁ ❁

You can find images of our collages in the wild on Instagram @feminist_collages_pgh.

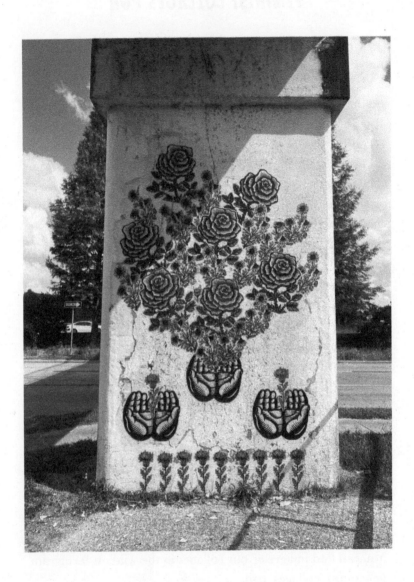

# KILL JOY

I was part of a community paste-up mural project to honor George Floyd in his childhood Third Ward neighborhood in Houston on the one-year anniversary of his murder. The next day, I used the leftover glue to create the wall pictured here using screen-printed versions of 5"x5" woodcut prints. It addresses the lack of clean air and water, healthy food, health care, affordable housing, and other basic necessities for a dignified life in my neighborhood, inhabited primarily by Latines.

I consistently find that in my community-fueled projects in Texas, and throughout Mexico and the Philippines, the most marginalized groups are most successfully organized by everyday women: mothers, teachers, peasant farmers, and neighbors. Women are not only demanding updated water drainage in our older neighborhoods prone to flooding during hurricanes but also building houses when homes are destroyed, organizing bulk meals for children whose families have little resources, and defending the land that they till and sow. As a BIPOC femme feminist, I'm in solidarity with women of the world who prioritize making life fuller and sweeter and bringing so much love to our neighborhoods.

❊   ❊   ❊

Kill Joy's work is grounded in honoring the earth and seeking environmental and social justice. She is an anarchist, artist, and cultural organizer who works in print, mural, and large-scale political puppets based in the US South. Her work can be seen on Instagram @kill.joy.land and Justseeds.org.

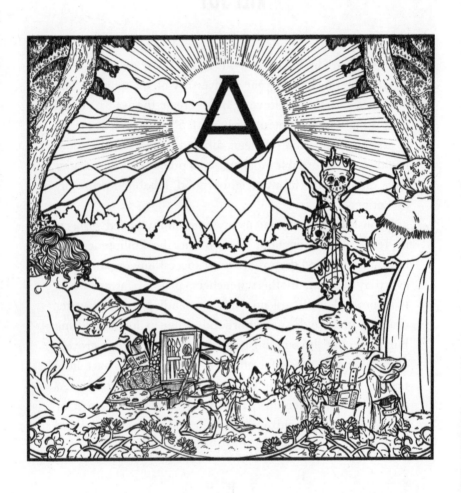

# N.O. BONZO

I frequently don't have a goal or specific statement I wish to convey with a piece other than enjoying the process. I understand anarchism as a distinct movement and identification that many have made incredible contributions to and sacrifices within. More often when I work, I think of people I know and those who've left memories of themselves behind. And for those who aren't here with us anymore, I reflect on how much we lose with their absence.

In this image, I thought of the black thread that's woven through generations, connecting us beyond walls, borders, states, and nationalities. Tracing that black thread shows how the beautiful idea itself forever reemerges in spite of countless rounds of violent repression against its adherents. I spend a lot of time these days trying to trace the black threads back, and become lost in the myriad stories of profound losses and victories of people hunted, tortured, and driven, yet still managing incredible feats, their hearts filled with their ideas. How one anarchist is able to sow the seeds from which a hundred spring up, even if it is decades later. And I think on them and us, and what we can contribute for future generations to carry in their hearts.

❊ ❊ ❊

N.O. Bonzo is an anarchist illustrator and printer. You can find them on Instagram @nobonzo and https://kolektiva. social/@nobonzo.

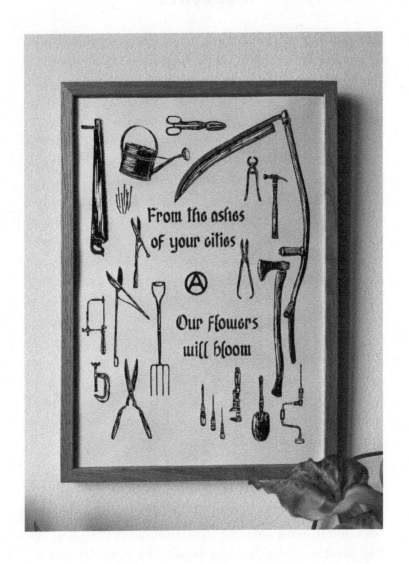

# RAYAN

The first thoughts I have every morning on waking are thoughts of anger—toward the human impact on nature and animals, and the general human need to dominate and destroy everything. That daily anger motivates me, gives me a sense of purpose, and even fills me with hope. So after a series of racist and queerphobic attacks in the big city where I currently reside, I created this print, composed of old farming tools that I've seen my grandmother use. These tools are sometimes sharp and can have a menacing appeal to them, but they can also connect us to the soil beneath our feet, helping us to survive and thrive with nature.

To be a feminist is to be against domination. Abolishing all sorts of human domination will be the fruit of our common labor, utilizing shared tools. Meaning at the end of the day when I close my eyes to imagine the beautiful world that we can create with each other, I see us blooming in it, together.

❊ ❊ ❊

Rayan's printmaking path started during the 2020 COVID confinement when aiming to raise money for animal sanctuaries. Their work then evolved into bigger-scaled prints while still tackling themes of anarchism, mutual aid, and ecology, all in the continuous hope of fundraising for projects they hold close to their heart. You can find Rayan on Instagram @rayan.forestgreen.

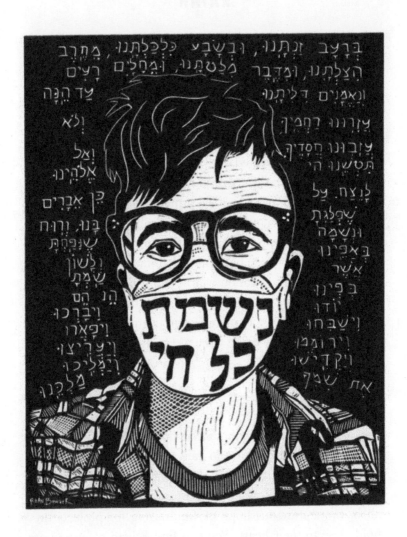

# ROAN BOUCHER

In this time of COVID, climate change, wildfires, and mass abandonment, I'm constantly thinking about breath and air as a source of life and sometimes harm—something that physically connects us all. Jewish liturgy is filled with references to *breath*, a word that in Hebrew also means "soul"; the words on the N95 in this print read "nishmat kol chai" (the breath/soul of every living being), and the words around it are from the same prayer. Throughout the pandemic, I've found ways to pray, sing, protest, organize, celebrate, and grieve collectively, with accessibility and COVID precautions centered, to keep our shared breath from causing injury. This is fundamental to the values of collective care, solidarity, consent, mutual aid, and liberation that I share with my communities, but that radicals broadly have often neglected.

In my art, I'm always thinking about these values and the emotions that go with them: joy, grief, and rage; sacredness, resilience, and beauty, and despair. Our connectedness is everything, whether we acknowledge it or not, whether we feel it or not. May we wake from the collective trance of individualism. May we keep each other safe, together, and make a new world that we can all live in.

❋ ❋ ❋

Roan Boucher is a trans Jewish artist and facilitator for social movement organizations. He makes art about queers, Judaism, movements, and liberation. His art can be found at roanboucher.com and on Instagram @pollinator_press_art.

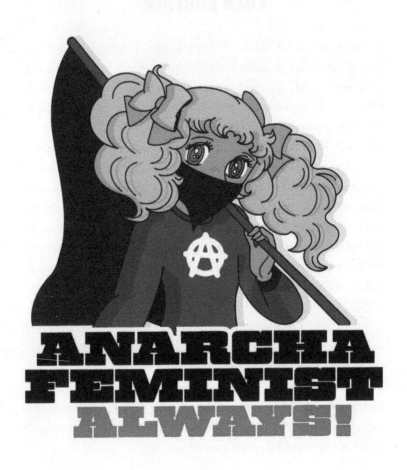

# SUGARBOMBING WORLD

I grew up watching Japanese anime. The first one I ever saw was *Candy Candy*, a normatively romantic, soap opera-style cartoon where patriarchal values, gender roles, and white beauty standards were everywhere. I always loved the drawings, but I could never get through an entire episode because of such messages. Through my own art, now as an adult, I've been able to reconnect with the type of cartoon I would've loved to watch as a kid, but I've subverted the character Candy, a blond girl, into a badass brown anarcha-feminist with rainbow hair.

During my artistic journey, I've found a lot of satisfaction in switching the gender roles that the media typically imposes on us. I even created a genre for this, which I call Subversive Pop. As some of my pieces proclaim, "We deserve a world that does not hurt," and that includes not only destroying patriarchy and protecting trans, queer, and femme folks, not only raising our black flags and fists against their violence, laws, and stereotypes, but also proudly and playfully showing that our feminism is anarchist or it isn't feminist at all.

❀ ❀ ❀

You can find more of Sugarbombing World's DIY art projects and no-border, fuck-the-police politics at https://sugarbombing-store.myshopify.com/ or on Instagram @sugarbombingworld.

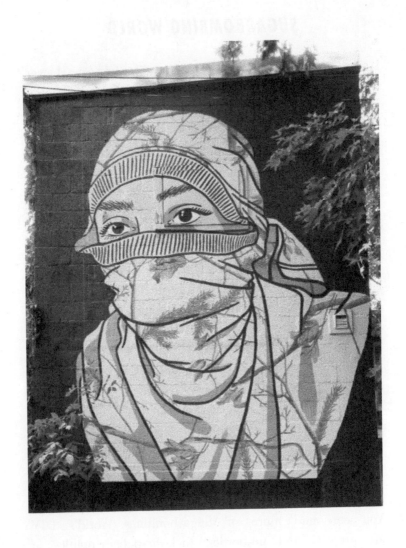

# ZOLA

This mural, done in 2022 in so-called Montreal, honors all nature, land, and forest defenders across the continent, battling capitalist tyrants to save what's left of the living world. I painted it thinking of frontline struggles such as Ada'itsx / Fairy Creek, Weelaunee forest in Atlanta, and Wet'suwet'en Yintah. With the accelerated encroachment on what remains of natural habitats, fighting to defend nature equates with fighting for humanity. I also used a pink realtree camo pattern to represent queer bush counterculture. Marginalized, gender-nonconforming people and freaks show up in numbers at land defenses. Because of our dysphoric experience with normative lifestyles, we see through the illusory comfort and false promises of "progress" in our capitalist hellscape. We see death creeping around the corner and find comfort in mutual relations between all ways of life.

As a militant, feminism is a methodology that drives me to be vulnerable with my peers and make sure to leave no one behind. As an artist, feminism inspires me to represent and uplift the experiences of people in resistance to patriarchy who are both brave and caring.

❖ ❖ ❖

Zola is a queer, settler anarchist and street artist up to no good, based in Montreal. Their wheat-pasted characters of rioters and anonymous protesters advocate for militancy, direct action, and unapologetic radical politics. You can find them, among other places, on Instagram @zola_mtl and Mastodon at kolektiva.social/@zola.

# REMEMBRANCE AND SUBVERSIVE BODIES IN MOTION

/

BREE BUSK

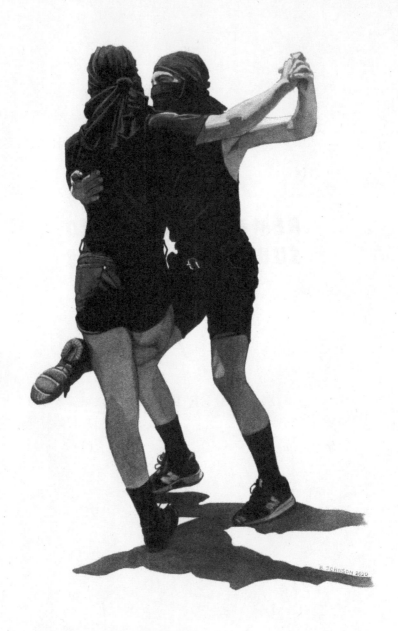

My compañera Karina once told me that it's a mistake to try to re-create the past. We were talking about the bittersweet sensation of looking back on the *estallido social* (social outbreak), the anti-neoliberal revolt that rippled through Chile in late 2019.[1] It left an indelible mark on those of us who lived through it, and not always metaphorically. While some came away with commemorative tattoos, others were left scarred or even maimed by tear gas canisters and crowd control rounds. Thirty-four people didn't come away at all. Despite the rage and horror, for many of us relatively young protesters— Chilean, Indigenous, or migrant—participating in that mass uprising dramatically transformed our understanding of what type of change was possible in our lifetimes.

Over three years have passed since that historic upending of business as usual, and we have undeniably entered darker times. The dream of the revolt—to overthrow the neoliberal system imposed during the dictatorship of Augusto Pinochet, and put an end to impunity and state violence in all of its forms—feels more unreachable than ever. In 2020, the Constitutional Convention became the primary vehicle for the broad spectrum of social demands raised during the protests—demands developed over the course of thirty years since Chile began its transition back to democracy, and channeled by the recent waves of student and feminist activism. When the proposed draft was voted down in the September 2022 plebiscite, a deep malaise spread through the country's left-wing social movements.

---

1. *Social outbreak* is the most commonly used term to describe this uprising, but those who participated and still align themselves with its goals often refer to it as *la revuelta* (the revolt).

Today, we're still deep in the *plebitusa*: a portmanteau that originated in Colombia in the wake of the 2016 Peace Accord to describe post-plebiscite disaffection. The proposed new constitution—globally acclaimed for its pro-democracy, feminist, environmentalist, and pro-Indigenous priorities—was meant to be our consolation prize after the pandemic consumed the momentum of our street protests. The proposal was ultimately pronounced dead on arrival, rejected by a majority driven into the arms of the Far Right by a fake news campaign that exacerbated people's anxiety over losing what little they had to so-called migrant invaders, degenerate Communists, or Indigenous terrorist cells.

On the Left, there was plenty of blame to go around, and in some cases, we were happy to turn on each other for bothering to have hope in the first place. I recently stumbled on a piece of Banksy-esque street art featuring two skeletons collapsed on the ground, holding signs inscribed with two of the most iconic slogans of the revolt: "Con todo si no pa' qué?" (Give it all, or why bother?) and "Hasta que la dignidad se haga costumbre" (Until dignity becomes the norm). As I trudged past, I wondered whether the artist intended the work to function as a reflection or accusation. Was the revolt symbolically murdered by the devastation of the pandemic or did it die of neglect when we directed our efforts toward the constitutional process? When a political moment has passed, what remains?

❊　❊　❊

The ghost of the revolt continues to haunt downtown Santiago in the form of graffiti slogans and tattered posters calling for the release of the remaining political prisoners. Mobile street vendors are still hawking flags, T-shirts, illustrations, art books, and glossy photographs featuring the most memorable faces and scenes of the revolt. The images persist even as the reality fades.

Chilean protests and protesters have an international reputation for being photogenic, even in our worst moments. There are the heroic *secundaries* (high schoolers) who are regularly documented dodging riot police, chucking molotovs, and romantically clutching hands in the midst of swirling clouds of tear gas. With the arrival of a new feminist wave in 2015 came topless university students sporting body paint and ostentatiously decorated balaclavas. And there is always the fire, creeping out of the smashed-in door of a bank, roaring up from a bonfire of trash and construction debris, or tracing the contour of a barricade blocking a major avenue. Even our pain and despair have an aesthetic dimension because there is always an army of professional photographers at the ready to document the brutality of the armed forces and bloody injuries that follow. There is little that goes undocumented, for better or worse.

At the dawn of 2023, these types of thrilling mass mobilizations have decreased in both number and frequency. The police repression—reaching shocking levels of violence at the height of the revolt—has persisted, surviving the transition to a so-called left-wing government a year earlier. The administration of Gabriel Boric was meant to be yet another consolation prize, a lesser evil who shone like a beacon in comparison with José Antonio Kast, his fascist opposition. I suppose it helps that we never expected much from him. And yet, as the joke goes, he still managed to disappoint us. Boric is currently overseeing the development of a new constitutional process—one carefully engineered to limit democratic participation and exclude the historical Indigenous and social movement demands introduced during the previous Constitutional Convention. People said "Chile despertó" (Chile woke up) in October 2019, but today it's that handful of months where the government was running scared that feels like a dream.

As an anarchist raised and radicalized in the United States, I think I've adapted to our bleak new reality a bit faster than my *compañeres*. I cut my teeth on the US antiwar movement of the mid-2000s, and the result of that struggle taught me that failure was the rule, not the exception. I had grown into my politics obsessing over an idealized past, dreaming of the Spanish Civil War because I couldn't imagine myself as an agent of change in the time and place I had been born into. I never expected to make history, first as part of an unprecedented anticapitalist feminist uprising in 2018 and again in 2019 in the massive revolt it fed into. After so many years of feeling powerless and outnumbered in my birth country, I will never forget what it was like to finally have a taste of *poder popular*.[2] It would be easy to turn the revolt into just another anarchist fantasy, one I can only return to

---

2. Poder popular (popular or people power) is a form of workers' or direct democracy. In Chilean history, it has referenced a form of political power derived from the independent activity of working-class people, which in its formulation and constitution is (in theory) highly collective, flexible, representative, and direct.

in dreams, but after nearly eight years living and fighting in Chile, I'm not as American as I used to be—that is to say, not as *estadounidense*.[3]

In Chile, remembrance is not synonymous with mere yearning for what has been lost. It is an act of resistance and our inheritance from the generation of people who resisted the dictatorship, often at the cost of their lives. I arrived in Santiago in August 2015, just in time to participate in the annual commemoration of the coup that took place on September 11, 1973. My compañera Romina took me to the National Stadium, a mass torture and detention site under the dictatorship that has since been converted into a site of memory. The stadium's facade was papered with posters featuring silhouettes and the refrain that has echoed throughout this country for fifty years: "¿Dondé están?" (Where are they?).

The names of the detained and disappeared, not to mention those whose lives were lost or stolen under democracy, haven't been forgotten. Thanks to the work of the feminist movement, this practice of commemoration extends to victims of femicide as well, including women who were murdered by the armed forces or extractive industries. When a martyr's or victim's name is cried out in any march or protest, a chorus of a hundred voices will answer "¡Presente!"—a callback that is both acknowledgment and battle cry.

We lit candles and toured the interior spaces that had once served as cells, pausing to listen to a crowd boisterously singing "Venceremos," the hymn of Salvador Allende's Popular

---

3. South Americans consider all the people of the Americas to be *americana/os*. I'm thus still "American," but no longer consider myself so bound to the United States in my political thinking or culture.

Unity coalition. The sound reverberated through the concrete corridors of the stadium, encouraging the singers to up the volume with every chorus. While some younger faces could be found in the crowd, it was clear that many of them were of an age to have fought for mass social and economic transformation in the 1960s and early 1970s, only to see their utopian dreams crushed under the boot of the military dictatorship. During his rule, Pinochet did everything in his power not only to wipe out any wisp of resistance but also destroy memory itself, hoping that no one would recall what it was like to live any other way. And yet people survived, and they hadn't forgotten how to sing.

The ongoing resistance of our political predecessors is a reminder that it is still possible to rediscover hope after a massive defeat, even when so much has been lost and fascism is once again on the rise. We are still collectively fumbling in the dark, searching for the exit from the *plebitusa*, and I suspect that in order to find our way back to the light, we will need to reengage with the revolt and its legacy, not as an idealized past to which we wish to return, but as one more red thread of rebellion that anchors our current, seemingly hopeless present to our own history of resistance, and one that also stretches forward into the future where an inevitable, irresistible revolution awaits us if only we keep building toward it.

❀ ❀ ❀

I have never wanted to write my *estallido* social story. At first, there was no need. I was experiencing something transcendent alongside millions of others. We didn't need to talk about it because we were living it. During the protests, marches, and countless other gatherings, I remember how easy it was to strike up a conversation with strangers or even just exchange complicit smiles. Our story was being told all over the world, through news reports, solidarity protests, art, and performance, and I was lost in the joyful collectivity of it all. In my own barrio, I followed the sound of banging pots and pans to a group of neighbors with whom I went on to form a popular assembly. Everything was special, but nothing was unique.

Today, my reasons are different. I don't think I'm alone in finding it difficult to think back on the good times from the perspective of the present. Even the walls of Santiago—historically a living record of the political upheavals of the day—have surprisingly little to say. The city is buffed with sloppy rectangles of gray paint—the right-wing answer to our colorful, positive propaganda. In 2022, street-level fascist groups had rediscovered the dictatorship era practice of painting over leftist or otherwise subversive posters and graffiti, and the result is a city with its history redacted. They want us to forget, which makes it so much more important for us to remember.

When I walk downtown, my memory is there to fill in the gaps left on the walls. As a member of the Brigada Laura Rodig, the feminist art and propaganda brigade of the Coordinadora Feminista 8 de Marzo (CF8M), I can narrate the revolt through an account of our political interventions.

Here, we painted a massive green *pañuelo* (bandana) bearing the slogan, "This government rapes, kills, and makes people disappear." There, on that wall, we plastered our mosaic portraits of movement martyrs as dirty wheat paste dripped into our eyes and hair. And here, on this corner, we tied red paper flowers to the fencing cordoning off the site where a protester fell to his death through an unsecured maintenance panel. Memories of these actions are frequently interspersed with personal ones. Watching roaming squads of hundreds of high school students break into the subway stations barricaded against them. Being ecstatically crushed among millions of protesters during "Chile's Biggest March." Witnessing the arrival of Las Tesis's iconic feminist performance "A Rapist in Your Path" to Plaza Dignidad (Dignity Square), the epicenter of the protests. I snapped photos of it all with my outdated smartphone, knowing that I would someday need to look back at it and remind myself it was real.

❊ ❊ ❊

It was November 23, 2019, and I was having the best day of my life. The revolt was in full swing, and I remember the ethereal quality of simply existing in public and seeing it unfold around me.

The historic Communist mural brigade, the Brigada Ramona Parra (BRP), had put out an open call for volunteers to join it in painting a massive mural alongside the Mapocho River where it passes Plaza Dignidad, and my compañera Denisse and I had decided it was an opportunity not to be missed. While neither of us had ever been attracted to the politics of the Chilean Communist Party, we had tackled similar public art projects as part of the Brigada Laura Rodig and were captivated by the idea of doing a collaborative mural on such a large scale. That was the official line, at least. If pressed, I would have had to admit to being a longtime BRP fangirl dying to see how my own street art skills measured up against those of the iconic *muralistas*.

I arrived early in the day and had a truly hair-raising experience descending a rickety ladder to the otherwise inaccessible riverbank. Strangers caught first my backpack and then me, as I tumbled from the final rungs. I was eventually joined by Denisse and dozens of other volunteers—some with experience, and others only with enthusiasm. The revolt was only a month old at that point, and there was a widespread feeling of entitlement to public space. The walls and streets were ours, and they would be the record of both our recent advances and revolutionary aspirations. We traced and painted the symbols that we all already recognized as part of the story we were writing together. A high school student jumping a turnstile. The infamous riot dog Matapacos and his red bandana. A masked protester. A grandmother wielding a wooden spoon to *cacerolear*—the action of beating on pots and pans as a form of popular protest. Dozens of eyes crying bloody tears, in acknowledgment of those who had recently been maimed by the police through their indiscriminate use of crowd control rounds. The mural was impossibly long, stretching out far beyond my line of sight. As I perched on a piece of scaffolding, paintbrush in hand, I felt the fleeting euphoria of what it was to be a part of history and wished it could last forever.

It didn't, of course, and it wasn't any easier on my way back up the ladder. I was sweaty and sunburned, but the thrill of the experience helped me push through my exhaustion. From the street, I could see other volunteers still working away on the mural's details. For anyone crossing the nearby bridge, it would be impossible to ignore.

It was early afternoon, and as I was essentially already at Plaza Dignidad, I thought I would take a walk around the area before going home. I was hoping to take photos of any new graffiti or posters that had appeared since the latest round of Friday night mobilizations. I began the lengthy process of crossing the multiple lanes of traffic that divided the river to the north from the plaza to the south. As I arrived at the final crosswalk, I encountered a hastily assembled barricade of construction debris that presented just enough of an obstacle to keep the oncoming traffic at bay. Music surged from a portable amplifier as a pair of masked tango dancers embraced in the middle of the street. The two of them moved as if they were the only couple left on earth, executing their graceful steps without a care for the growing threat from the drivers who tapped their horns in irritation. Each movement was timed to perfection, demonstrating both passion and athleticism. It was a performance that would have looked at home on any stage, but contained many layers of carefully considered symbolism.

The dancers wore matching black shirts and shorts with T-shirts tied over their faces in the style employed by protesters of all ideologies (not to mention the young, apolitical, angry, and disaffected) disposed to engaging in direct combat with the police. Their fitted clothing and lithe, queer-coded bodies were in stark contrast, however, with those of the stereotypical cis male rock-throwers who often wore typical street clothes or simply stripped down to their shorts, sneakers, and bandanas.

The choice of music also struck me; I recognized the sound of La Lira Libertaria, a local group known for drawing on the popular musical and poetry traditions of the region to interpret modern antiauthoritarian themes. Years earlier, my friend Vicky had insisted on introducing me to their music as part of a crash course in what it meant to be a Chilean anarchist. The dancers had choreographed their tango to "Ármate," a song that begins as a melancholy ballad, but builds to a chorus that demands listeners to "arm yourself and be violent, beautifully violent," a phrase recalling the words of Luisa Toledo, a beloved revolutionary icon of resistance against the dictatorship who relentlessly championed the creative, destructive power of young people until her death in 2021.

Felipe and Manuel, I would later learn, were professional dancers who performed as Zuinger, a duo committed to breaking the gender binary as well as bringing their queer take on traditional dance out of the studio and into public space. In the short documentary film *Sentido y razón* by Martín Pizarro Veglia, Felipe describes Chile as a country in which everything is oriented around the cisgender male gaze. Where, they wonder, is there room for women, queers, and transgender people?[4] At first, like so many other broke and talented young people, the duo performed along the busy sidewalks of downtown Santiago in exchange for tips. When the October uprising overtook the capital, they made

4. *Sentido y razón*, written and directed by Martín Pizarro Veglia (Chile, 2021), 19 min., https://cinechile.cl/pelicula/sentido-y-razon/.

the decision to take Zuinger to Plaza Dignidad, where they performed in the midst of tear gas and water cannons. And that is where I encountered them, claiming space for those of us who burned to bring our liberated bodies out into the streets and be "beautifully violent" ourselves.

A small crowd had gathered to watch the performance that day, and as motorists tried to nudge their way past the barricade, we nonchalantly blocked the gaps with our bodies and whatever else came to hand. No words were spoken; none were needed. The plaza had been ours for weeks, and we were the ones to decide how it—and indeed public space all over the country—would be used going forward. As I watched, I snapped photos and thought, "I am finally living in the new world we have fought for. In this world, beautiful, unexpected things will be the rule, not the exception."

❖ ❖ ❖

In the first weeks of the pandemic, I suddenly had more time on my hands than I knew what to do with. Although I still considered myself a painter, I had largely abandoned my personal practice in favor of collective projects and the capitalist grind. The quarantine was almost a blessing in that sense; at last, I could look back on my collection of photos from a busy year of protests and select the best to use as painting references. Even then, I think I understood that the pandemic meant the end of the revolt as I knew it, but I still anticipated the idea of returning to those memories with pleasure, knowing that the act of painting was a way to escape my dull, uncertain present.

I chose a photo I had taken of the tango dancers, of course. Not only did they make for an objectively stunning subject, but I felt compelled to put the feeling I had that day into a painting. For me, creating art is a type of meditation. As a practitioner of photorealism, I spend days and sometimes weeks concentrating on every line and shadow. I come to know my subjects intimately. And whether I am painting a comrade or an anonymous muse, it is always an act of love.

Given that we're living in historic times, I think it is also my way of giving weight and importance to what I think is worth remembering. My comrades are worth remembering, as are the activities we've organized together. The spontaneous acts of beauty and resistance I've witnessed are worth remembering too. I don't see myself as an individual artist distantly recording events as they unfold but rather a participant in the project of building our collective memory of this period—a record not only of what passed but also what it meant to us and how it felt to live through it.

When I completed my painting, *El Tango Encapuchao (The Masked-Up Tango)*, and shared it on social media, I received some positive feedback from friends and fans who in turn shared it with their own networks. A few days later, I was shocked to receive a message from Felipe, one of the dancers depicted in the painting. Through a series of audio messages, they told me that seeing the painting had truly moved them and they couldn't thank me enough for creating it. Once the pandemic was over, we promised each other that we would sit down together for a coffee and indulge in a little mutual admiration. I mentioned my dream of exhibiting my quarantine era paintings someday, and Felipe immediately committed to performing at the opening. Although the possibility of having a public event seemed so distant, it went straight to my heart that someone who had inspired me so much could in turn take something from my own art; that neither the performance nor my photo nor even the painting itself would be the end of this cycle.

Nearly two and a half years later, in October 2022, the exhibition finally became a reality. I had sent a proposal to the collective that managed Librería Proyección, the beloved radical bookstore and infoshop where I attended so many meetings and other activities, and it had agreed to host my exhibition, including an opening night. After so much time spent in lockdown, I was eager to turn the event into something of a coming out, a return to the streets. I was still in mourning over the shocking defeat of the proposed new constitution one month earlier, but as the slogan goes, it "smelled like October"—the month the revolt had kicked off—and my rebellious heart was waking back up.

Once the date was set, the first thing I did was write to Felipe. Part of me expected them to have forgotten their promise, but they instantly reassured me that they wouldn't miss my opening night for the world. While their former dance partner, Manuel, had moved to Spain, Felipe informed me that they were now working with a new partner, Rodrigo, who would be pleased to perform. With that crucial detail squared away, I shifted my thoughts to how I could bring my exhibition out of the gallery and into public space.

I decided to create a *gigantografía*, a popular form of street art I'd learned about alongside my compañeras at the height of the feminist wave. I used a free internet program to transform a digital scan of *El Tango Encapuchao* into a ninety-one-page PDF, which I then printed out and laboriously pasted together on my living room floor. The result was a mosaic poster nearly twice my height, ready to be pasted onto a wall of my choosing. After some discussion with my contact at the bookstore about logistics, I set my sights on a blank wall just north of the entrance.

The day of the exhibition, I put out a call within my feminist organization for extra hands. A handful of compañeras showed up just in time to help, and to my surprise, Felipe and Rodrigo arrived early for their rehearsal and decided to pitch in. Together, we scrubbed the wall clean and began the arduous work of wheat pasting the poster high above our heads, out of reach of passing fascists and their buckets of gray paint. Rodrigo was the most fearless, using his dancer's grace to balance on the highest rungs. Felipe and I couldn't stop smiling at each other as we worked, and after all, why not? Foot by messy foot, we were reintroducing their performance—so grounded in another place and time—to our post-plebiscite reality.

When we had finally achieved our goal and stepped back to admire our work, we all grinned for selfies and squeezed each other's hands in excitement. Nearly two weeks prior to the second anniversary of the revolt, we had made something new that was neither a melancholic commemoration nor a nostalgic commodity. It was street art in its best sense, done without permission by comrades old and new, dragging hope back out of our mourning and pasting it up on a wall for the world to see.

I left the dancers outside to rehearse and returned to the work of preparing the exhibition. I moved chairs, straightened frames, and scrubbed my face clean of the soot that had rained down on us while we worked. A short time later, I began welcoming my guests, nearly all of whom were compañeras of my own organization or friends from our broader activist community. When it was time for me to speak, I talked about how it still hurt to think back on the revolt and how I had worried that my art, a record of my own experiences, would end up as just another cynical commodification of something priceless. And then I told the story of the best day of my life and the painting that commemorates it, and how it's helped me pick up the thread of rebellion again and again. It meant everything to me that something so beautiful and profound could keep growing from one October to the next and find new life even in this difficult new era, when we need it the most. I was met with hugs and tears and words of support from my dear community, which I am pleased to say, had no idea what was coming next.

My compañera Fernanda, the MC for the event, corralled us all out of the bookstore and onto the large paved area in front of the building. High above and to the right of our small crowd, the gigantografía was gloriously visible, shining out from the drab bricks and concrete of downtown Santiago. And then the music started, and I didn't have eyes for anything else but the long, elegant leg emerging from the bookstore entrance. As Felipe and Rodrigo executed their first steps, all in black, T-shirts wrapped around their faces, moving with all the exquisite passion that the tango has to offer, I finally felt it again: that same surging joy I remembered from when I first saw two dancers come together to perform behind a barricade.

And I realized what should have been obvious all along. It has always been our queer, feminist, subversive bodies in motion—mourning, remembering, and resisting—that are the ultimate legacy, not only of the revolt, but of all revolts. For those of us who are still here, the stories we have lived will be the memory of resistance for those who come next.

Los años siguen su rumbo y el olvido no descansa
Volviendo la vida mansa, dejándola sin memoria
Burlando su trayectoria, ya que así el poder avanza
Más nos queda y el incendio al que me apego
Volviendo el recuerdo al fuego que como plaga se expande
Porque ante todo el que mande no seré nunca borrego

The years march on and oblivion doesn't rest
Making life tame, stripping it of memory
Twisting its course, since that's how power advances
More remains for us and the blaze I cling to
Turning memory back into a fire that spreads like a plague
Because in the face of any authority, I will never be a follower

—La Lira Libertaria, "Ármate"

❉   ❉   ❉

Bree Busk is an anarchist, writer, and artist based in Santiago, where she discovered her true political home during the 2018 feminist uprising. Her art can be found on Instagram @breeatlast, and her collected writing and interviews can befound at linktr.ee/breeatlast. Thanks goes out to Felipe, Manuel, and Rodrigo as well as all of Bree's CF8M compañeras, who have been simultaneously the most tireless supporters of her work and her greatest sources of inspiration.

# SHAKESQUEER TUCSON: PERFORMING ANARCHO-FEMINISM

/

WREN AWRY

On a Friday evening in April 2022, in the street in front of autonomous social center BCC Tucson, a figure crept out of the shadows and onto a hand-painted stage.[1] "In fair Verona where we lay our scene," the Chorus began, and with this invocation, Shakesqueer's production of *Romeo and Juliet* commenced. But it wasn't a straightforward version of the play: Verona was depicted as an egalitarian commune tucked in a crystal abyss, Romeo and Juliet were both queer women, and the people of Verona were fed up with the squabbling Montague and Capulet families, which were still holding onto their wealth and power. Over the next three hours, romance and intrigue erupted across the stage, lit in soft neon shades, and filled with actors draped in metallic chains and white lace.

*Romeo and Juliet* was the fourth production of Shakesqueer, an all-volunteer crew in Tucson, Arizona, that puts on queer, radical interpretations of the Bard's work. Throughout the course of the 2022 spring season—during rehearsals for the play and after it was done—I interviewed members of Shakesqueer about the troupe, and the ways in which these performances create a community of care while striving to embody queer, feminist, and anarchist ideals.[2] What follows is an informal oral history, stitched together from bits and pieces of those conversations.

---

1. For more information on BCC Tucson, see https://bcctucson.org/.

2. I'm also a member of Shakesqueer, and have been part of *Macbeth* (2018), *As You Like It* (2019), and *Romeo and Juliet* (2022) in onstage and behind-the-scenes capacities. Since these interviews took place, Shakesqueer has put on a fifth production, *A Midsummer Night's Dream* (2023), also performed at BCC Tucson.

## CAST, IN ORDER OF APPEARANCE

**Maggie Dwenger:** *Twelfth Night* (director and Malvolio), *Macbeth* (Macduff and logistics), *As You Like It* (Touchstone), and *Romeo and Juliet*, 2020 and 2022 (Juliet and media)[3]

**Glen Frieden:** *Twelfth Night* (director and narrator), *Macbeth* (Lady Macbeth), *As You Like It* (Jacques and stage manager), and *Romeo and Juliet*, 2020 and 2022 (Juliet's nurse and acting coaching)

**Ember Buck:** *Twelfth Night* (Maria), *Macbeth* (codirector), *As You Like It* (Rosalind/Ganymede), and *Romeo and Juliet*, 2020 (assistant director and Lady Capulet)

**Inmn Neruin:** *Macbeth* (Banquo and prop fabrication), *As You Like It* (codirector, cowriter, Phebe, and Charles the Wrestler), *Romeo and Juliet*, 2020 (Mercutio), and *Romeo and Juliet*, 2022 (director, Gregory, and Apothecary)

**Sophie Maloney:** *As You Like It* (Duke Frederick and Audrey), *Romeo and Juliet*, 2020 (Balthasar and technical director), and *Romeo and Juliet*, 2022 (Mercutio and technical director)

---

3. One week before *Romeo and Juliet* was scheduled to open in March 2020, it was canceled due to the COVID-19 pandemic. The production was directed by Adrian Provenzano and had a somewhat different cast, although many of the same elements, including the stage, were used in 2022. Throughout our conversations, those who were part of the 2020 production emphasized the importance of naming and acknowledging the first iteration, since so much work and creativity went into it.

**Dominique Gualaman:** *Romeo and Juliet*, 2022 (Romeo and miscellaneous support)

**Egg:** *Romeo and Juliet*, 2022 (Tybalt and miscellaneous support)

**Adrian Provenzano:** *Twelfth Night* (Viola), *Macbeth* (Malcolm), *As You Like It* (Silvius, Amiens Family Band member, and puppetry), *Romeo and Juliet*, 2020 (director), and *Romeo and Juliet*, 2022 (Chorus and costume coordinator)

## ACT 1: "WE COULD JUST PUT ON A PLAY WITH OUR FRIENDS"

**Maggie:** I was unemployed at the time. Glen had just moved to town, and I was trying to engage him as a new friend. I knew that he had community theater experience. I was like, "That's so funny, because I have no experience whatsoever. But I love Shakespeare. And I have a lot of time on my hands." I thought it might work because Tucson was this place where I saw a lot of people being active in cool ways. You're doing hard work with your friends, and it's actually producing something.

**Glen:** Yeah, we *could* do that! We could just put on a play with our friends.

**Ember:** At a release party for a No More Deaths abuse documentation report, Maggie and Glen said, "We're thinking about putting on a Shakespeare play."[4] That was my first full

---

4. No More Deaths aims to, in its own words, "end death and suffering in the Mexico-US borderlands through civil initiative." For more information, see https://nomoredeaths.org/en/.

year in Tucson, and one of the moments when I was like, "The fact that this came up without me even being the instigator of it means that I'm 100 percent in the correct community for me." Because one of my fondest memories from childhood is going to Shakespeare in the Park in Kansas City. The theater company would put on a Shakespeare summer camp, which I attended and loved.

**Glen:** Somebody suggested, "Glen and Maggie should direct." Then we sent out an email. The subject line was, "It wasn't a joke." We invited nine or ten of our closest friends in Tucson to a meeting. People we thought might be interested in it. At that meeting, we explained, "We're gonna do the play, we're gonna have rehearsals, we're gonna have auditions. Me and Maggie are gonna direct. Does this sound good to everybody?" We just kind of went for it.

**Inmn:** I got involved in Shakesqueer when I was living in Asheville, North Carolina, and I came to Tucson to help with the No More Deaths Spring Break. It was the first day that I got into town, and I ran into a friend, and they said, "Are you going to the play tonight?" They told me that this group was putting on a production of *Twelfth Night* and the theme was "space punk," and it was all genderbent and wacky. So I drove all the way down to Arivaca, Arizona, to catch the last performance and absolutely fell in love with it from the moment the curtains opened. Then the next year I was in town visiting in the winter again and got a random text message from a friend about auditions for *Macbeth*, a second production that Shakesqueer was putting on.

**Sophie:** I got involved in *As You Like It* just through word of mouth with friends. I had done theater stuff growing up and in high school. It was this really revolutionary concept to me that a group of friends could just be like, "We are going to do theater," and then be able to do that in an informal way.

**Dominique:** I saw *Macbeth* and loved it. I saw *As You Like It*. Loved it. Dressed up for *As You Like It*, in a flower crown and floral clothing and fun makeup. Tried to get others to participate via bringing more flowers to wear and saying, "Here's yours, here's yours, here's yours." I remember running lines with Ember because they were in *As You Like It*. When the auditions happened for the 2022 production of *Romeo and Juliet*, I actually wanted to play the Nurse for a fun thing to do. Glen encouraged me to try out for a bigger role, so I looked at some of the monologues and showed up to the audition semi-prepared and very much excited. And also excited to get the role of Romeo and terrified to get the role.

**Egg:** Someone I knew was in *As You Like It*. I went and saw it. I read the playbill that you probably wrote, Wren, and I was really excited because I had just read Silvia Federici's *Caliban and the Witch*, and thought, "Oh, all of this material about the enclosure of the commons is really doing it for me." I didn't follow Shakesqueer closely enough to be part of the first production of *Romeo and Juliet*, but when there was an open call for auditions in winter 2021, that's when I tried out.

## ACT 2: "NO ONE PERSON COULD HAVE POSSIBLY DREAMED UP WHAT IT IS"

**Adrian:** Because the majority of the people in the group every year have been radicals, or people who believe in revolution and liberation, that has influenced what we create. Even if we're not always going around and saying we're an anarcho-queer project or anarcho-feminist project, I think we're all people who are aware of power, people who are aware of control and hierarchies, and want to act on that in our smaller collectives that we create and form a different way of relating to one another. Because of that, we shift the plays to take out moments, or shift those moments to feel better in relation to what our ideals and values are.

Sometimes it's really in your face in a fun way, like at the end of *Macbeth*, killing me, the king, and yelling, "Never another king, never another cop, never another policeman, never another president," and blood foaming from my mouth. And then taking that on tour to rural Arizona was intense. We had to have conversations about what we felt was appropriate. I think we decided to not use all the same language when we were in Ajo. We had a whole consensus meeting about it. It's not that we wanted to censor ourselves but rather we asked, "What's appropriate in different spaces?"

**Egg:** Part of putting together a production that makes it have these elements of anarchism could be found in other theater productions as well, which is beautiful when you think about it. But the elements that make Shakesqueer anarchist are the ways in which the cast becomes mutually dependent on one another in the formation of this creative project; we rely on the work that we and our peers are putting into the endeavor. The other thing we do as a cast is to be deeply involved in the set creation and creative visioning of the project. There is no distinct line separating directors from other participants.

**Glen:** Anarchism, at least in my understanding, means the minimizing of hierarchy. And putting on a play is coordinating a sizable group of people into doing an extremely specific and predetermined set of actions. With this project, those hierarchies have always been put under the microscope of the group, or very, very much put out there in the group, such as, "This is what we're doing, we're thinking about creating a temporary, consensual hierarchy here." That to me is anarchist; when those top-down structures pop up, they can be disassembled by the group if they are not legitimate or whatever.

**Adrian:** We've had a couple of iterations of how much control the director did or did not have throughout the years. There's been moments when people feel like the director has too much control, and yet those plays went extremely smoothly. And then there's been moments when the directors have felt like they didn't want to have much control or power, and want it to be more consensual, and then it was a lot bumpier and slower and maybe a little more chaotic of a production. I feel like this past year, we hit a real sweet spot. Inmn had a vision and a real story that they wanted to tell. We all really loved that vision and story, and wanted to help create that story. But there were certain moments when Inmn wanted to do something and the rest of the cast didn't want to, and we did a consensus process and then Inmn's ideas didn't happen.

**Sophie:** I didn't really get exposed to collective and non-hierarchical organizing until coming to Tucson, and the Shakesqueer project has been one of those things that really has shown me how possible it is to organize and orient in that way. Sometimes it feels really messy, but especially with *As You Like It*, there's all of these ideas that came up where I was like, "That's impossible," or, "I don't know if that really fits with the rest of the play." And then watching all of those things actually manifest and happen in these beautiful, chaotic ways that then blended together, it was a really visible way of seeing how collective processes can work. How breaking down those power structures can bring about such cool art and creativity. No one person could have possibly dreamed up what it is.

**Dominique:** Toward the beginning of *Romeo and Juliet* rehearsals, we had a meeting specifically for what our COVID protocols were going to be. We were in the middle of a COVID wave again; it was in January. We were still masking at the rehearsals, and being outside and trying to keep distance and stuff like that. As the numbers went down, we relaxed some of those protocols. It felt good; we were trying to move through that according to what science and numbers showed us.

The decision on how the play was going to end was collaborative in a couple of different ways. We played with the idea of Juliet living, Juliet killing Paris, or maybe the play ending after Juliet stabs herself, and not having the families come and see Romeo and Juliet. That was all a group discussion. All of that collaboration is the anarcho side, and on the feminism side, I feel like some aspects of feminism are so basic, like let's just not have cis men in charge of everything.

Yet more than that, I feel like it's gearing toward the idea of what feminism could be when it's actualized.

**Egg:** I suppose the way that I see it as a feminist project is that the tasks of putting it together don't become sharply differentiated and the people taking them on are not stratified, not doing so because they are forced into a position of caretaking, cleaning up, or taking responsibility for things that others are avoiding because of a desire to be in the spotlight or do more glamorous tasks. It's kind of analogous in my mind to other autonomous projects where everyone does the dishes.

**Maggie:** In more subtle ways, I think Shakesqueer does reflect anarcho-feminism and anarcho-queerness by empowering people to take on creative projects that maybe they haven't had access to before. Along with all of that there's some sort of DIY aesthetic that I really love. I think it's so cool that with the first play, almost no one had theater experience. We worked through that together, and we trusted each other to put in the work to learn those skills and then share those skills with our community.

**Adrian:** The first year or maybe two years, we never called it Shakesqueer. But _Twelfth Night_ was an extremely queer production; we just didn't brand ourselves as queer. I think that reflects the fact that most of the members are queer, and we had a poly love fest at the end of _Twelfth Night_ where everyone got together and it was really fun.

**Ember:** I just started calling it Shakesqueer and put that on the posters for _Macbeth_. But there was definitely a misconception within the group after I did that that only queers could participate, whereas I had been much more of the opinion that we were queering Shakespeare. A queer reading of these texts, and then sometimes it's queer reinterpretation or remix and rewriting. Queer casting, of course. In mainstream theater, it's called "genderblind" casting, but that's too neutral for what we're doing. When I was casting for *Macbeth*, I was like, "I want some gay! I want some gay stuff going on!" So that's the opposite of gender-neutral casting. Queer was a part of it from the beginning, and it was really fun to tease out those elements from the text because they're already just right there.

**Egg:** I think that Shakespeare's writing already offers up a lot of space for queer possibility. In his plays as well as his other writing and sonnets, you can easily read how different forms of love are explored.

**Inmn:** *As You Like It* is about this "woman" who disguises herself as a man to travel about the world more easily and safely, and ends up meeting a man who's in love with her, but doesn't know that she is a her because she's disguised as a man and starts to court him as this man, which is very gay. That's just how the play originally is. But in the original version, she unveils at the end and can marry this man because she's actually a woman. In our version, which feels very familiar to me, through playing at being another gender, you can find the ways in which the gender that you've been raised in is not necessarily the gender that you are, the experience that you have, or the identity that you embody.

I remember being obsessed with reading about these female protagonists in stories. Then you know, later reflecting, "Did I have crushes on these characters? Or did I just want to be them?" and then realizing later that I just wanted to be them, that I was trans but didn't know it. So in our version of *As You Like It*, Rosalind, the woman who disguises herself as a man to navigate the world, in doing so realizes that they are not a woman. At the end of the play, they come out as being nonbinary trans. So the reveal at the end of *our* play was that they could marry everyone because they liked them all.

**Dominique:** There was queerness in a lot of different aspects of *Romeo and Juliet*. There was a story line of Mercutio having a big old crush on Romeo that was kind of unrequited; falling in love with your best friend, that does happen. We discussed early on, too, do we want part of Romeo and Juliet's star-crossed lovership to be that their parents are homophobic? And we decided no, we don't want that to be a part of this story because it's part of so many other stories and it's kind of overdone. Let's just have this in a queer utopia sense where that's actually not the issue at all.

The costumery had elements of, "What is gender?" even with Glen's role as the Nurse. There's a lot of roles that are "male," and the Nurse was not really one of them, but then Glen being the perfect Nurse, wearing the elements of a nurse and talking about being a wet nurse. Then there's a number of characters who use they/them pronouns. We're confined by some of the words, but we've changed some of the words to be what we want them to be. There was a fat joke in one of the exchanges, and I asked, "Can we take that out?" and the group replied, "Oh, yeah, strike it! Done!"

**Inmn:** In a few of the productions, we've tried to write in or amplify anarchistic ideals that are already present in the play or that we want to insert into the play to tell a certain story. In *As You Like It,* there's this historical footnote that the play was written in response to the Enclosure Act and enclosure riots. Even though it's this play in which nobility are some of the protagonists, they're nobility who've been exiled by this evil duke, and they go to live in the forests, and there's all of these jokes in the play that took me a really long time to decode that are about random farmers and sheep herders feeling weird about accepting wages for work. And then digging deeper into it and finding that this play was also written at a time when there was a shift going on from feudalism to early capitalism.

Seeing these small pieces of it in this play, whether it's nobles who no longer have feudal power going around and paying people to do things, and re-creating these structures through the exchange of money, or a bunch of people who have been exiled and are now hiding out in the forest, which was a huge part of the commons that were being encroached on and that ordinary people completely relied on to live. These were all parts of the play that were written into the original text, but were so subtly buried that to the nobility at the time it wouldn't have appeared to be this heavy critique of the shift into capitalism or feudal power structures, but a lot of common people would have gotten the jokes and references that were being made. So we amplified those footnotes and subtle references, and turned them into a larger backdrop in the play.

## ACT 3: "JOY ABSOLUTELY CONNECTS WITH CARE"

**Adrian:** I want to talk about the feelings of this play, *Romeo and Juliet*, in regard to care or mutual aid, which is an anarchist principle. We really came into that this year, where there was a lot of reciprocal care happening within the play. There was a lot of checking in and making sure people's needs were met, a lot of consensus process, asking people what they needed, and helping them get those things. In a lot of ways, it's a feminist ideal as well: making sure people in the collective have what they need and listening to people.

**Dominique:** If someone was having a stressful time in their personal life or because of the play, there was actual caring. I got stressed out because some of the content of the play was reigniting my work stressors [working as a nurse throughout the COVID-19 pandemic] and I wasn't fully mentally prepared for that to happen. I wasn't sure if I was gonna mention it, but then decided to talk with Inmn and Adrian about it. I talked to some other friends too, but within this group of new ones, I trusted that they would be kind and allow me some grace to kind of freak out.

**Maggie:** It's really hard to be vulnerable and do art with your friends. In order for that to actually happen, you have to create an atmosphere of care so that you can actually learn, mess up, play around, and do a lot of different things with acting. A lot of people struggle with public performances.

I was talking with Adrian, who was the director for the first round of *Romeo and Juliet*, about how I didn't feel like I had a lot of confidence in my acting and was struggling at rehearsals because I didn't think that I was doing it well. She sat me down and told me all the ways that I was able to generate emotion within her when I acted. It's such a confidence booster for your friends to see you grow in an art form and support you in that as well.

**Egg:** Care showed up as people taking collective and individual responsibility in the creation of the project as a whole, and care also showed up in many interpersonal dynamics that I was a part of and witnessed. Learning all the fight choreography for *Romeo and Juliet*, there were these moments of really embodied care when Dominique would knock me down, stand over me, and murder me during every practice, and then extend her hand and lift me up, pat me on the back, and wipe the dirt off me.

Another form that care took was in people encouraging one another to be the best that they could be. There was this moment midway through rehearsals when Glen spoke to the whole group, and as a reminder to people to memorize their lines, said, "If we had our lines memorized by now, we could all be focusing more on acting." It was a gentle invitation to the group that probably could have felt a little bit like shaming in a way, but instead was kind and helpful.

**Inmn:** Having been the director twice now and getting to work really closely with people on some of the acting stuff, it's been beautiful to watch people take on these roles or build intimacy with their scene partners in ways that they might not have ever done before. We're always all learning about the production while it's happening. One of our members always has some note about historical Shakespeare stuff to tell everyone at rehearsals or someone's like, "Wait, what does this word mean?" and then somebody knows the historical significance behind it.

Acting in general can provide this playful structure for people to participate in ways that they don't normally get to in their everyday life, to go and put on these other personas, and play around in them for a little while, maybe learn something new about themselves or their relationship to gender or any of the themes in the play. Watching people get to perform as villains, for instance, where they just have to be irrationally angry in ways that the actor maybe never really gets to play around with. I think there's a lot of potential for therapeutic healing that comes with putting on a production like this, especially in an environment where a lot of us are pretty amateur. There's room to explore stuff in ways that I hope feel less intimidating to people when they're not at some regular production worrying that the director's gonna yell at them for not remembering their lines or something.

**Dominique:** A couple of things were going wrong on the second night of *Romeo and Juliet*. Someone was mentioning the second night curse, and I was like, "What the fuck is that?" But definitely things were going wrong and awry. We had a little meeting in the intermission, and there was someone who had a slightly harsh tone, and someone else offered, "Come on. Let's be gentle with each other." That's a beautiful thing. That's a beautiful reminder.

**Ember:** Something that's amazing about theater is how immersive it is. It seems impossible to not get swept up in the primacy of the play—the play's the thing. Every play follows this arc, and toward the end, all of this momentum starts building and building and building. I've definitely seen, in lots of different kinds of productions that are building momentum, breaking points and tension explosions between folks, and also it's an amazing display of community. Because of that momentum, it's really, really hard to crap out on. Part of it is having a strong mutual goal that's also time bound. Putting those kinds of constraints on ourselves encourages us to figure out how to care for each other and problem solve. In some ways, the timing and pressure make a community of care necessary. Otherwise, it would be miserable, and we wouldn't keep doing it.

**Sophie:** A lot of our world is oriented by work and then activism. There have been times in my life where I feel like I just work and go to meetings. Shakesqueer was a huge thing for me of making and deepening friendships. I think when we're just meeting people at parties or something casually, we're not working or building something together in the same way. There's a magic to theater, especially doing shows and stuff; it's fun, exhilarating, and energizing, and that energy has this kind of social stickiness or glue to it that is really important for building community.

I've met people through that process who I'm now good friends with, and I feel more cared for overall in the community because I think we've been through stuff together, even if it's sort of fun-slash-stage-stress. This year there are new cast members; they're maybe not somebody I would have met or interacted with a lot, and thus get to form bonds with. It's nice to go to rehearsal and do something creative too. There's a huge community care aspect in that—saying this is worth our time to do and figure out.

**Maggie:** The first time we did a play, everyone in the audience didn't really understand what we were doing, and so when they saw it, they realized, "Oh, they're actually putting on a play and memorized the lines." It generated joy and love in the community for the coming days afterward and maybe even further. Why I love doing events in general is creating a space for the community to come together that's not always based around a party or something. How can we think through different things or show each other talents that maybe we don't usually show each other? Joy absolutely connects with care.

I was talking to Ember within the first couple years of doing Shakesqueer and said, "This is just fun work. It's not political work." And Ember was like, "Why is it not political work also? It's just a different kind of political work than we're used to." That really struck a chord with me: that political work is not always in the streets or on the border or whatever. Also, if you've done projects with your friends that take a lot of coordination and working together, what results is that you are better able to work together in the future on a diversity of projects. We fucked around and did rehearsals and a play for three months, and that made it so when we're doing, for example, Tucson Mesh or stuff with the BCC, it makes it that much easier to come at it trusting that you can do something with someone else and that you've had fun with that person.[5]

_____

5. Tucson Mesh is a community-controlled and collectively run wireless internet network that offers sliding-scale and low-cost internet access. For more information, see https://tucsonmesh.net/.

**Inmn:** It's always been really special to me that we have this commitment to going on small tours and bringing queer theater to rural places. Like going to Arivaca, which is this small town near the border, and bringing this production to this place where a lot of people, I think, don't really get to see anything like that very often. Or bringing it to Ajo, where one of our friends brought their middle school class to the production, and queer and trans kids in that class got to see this play that was very much put on for people like them. Or the ways that it offers collaboration between a lot of people; for instance, there's someone who has traditionally done a lot of the music for the play, and they bring an anarchistic brass band with them. It just turns into this big old production that a lot of people in the community have stakes and participation in.

**Maggie:** I don't think that we just do theater and everything's great. It's a specific way to tell stories, to bring community together, to build our ability to be creative together. It's just one part of many things that we can do together that creates a better world. It makes me sad to think about a project like Shakesqueer ending, but I think that it's OK for certain projects to come and do something special, and then they don't have to be institutionalized, you know? We should only be doing this if it's creating joy and happiness in our community. Let's stop when it's not doing that and let other people decide what they want to do.

## ACT 4: "WE'RE DEMONSTRATING SOMETHING TO OURSELVES BY DOING IT"

**Dominique:** The obvious potential is to fuck shit up, and with creativity, destroy the harmful structures of society within this little space that we're creating. For a moment, for a night, for a few hours, queerness isn't the issue; for a few hours this element of friendship and magic and crystals and all of that can exist. I used to play the strings for this country band that sang songs about being gay. We played gay bars in small towns in the Midwest and Southeast, or we played smaller venues. It's a similar feeling of, "For this time, in this room, we are going to create the world that we want to live in." My hope is that people get so invigorated, recharged, and inspired by that feeling that we all created for the audience that they go and do it themselves in their lives. It exponentially makes more spaces where that can exist.

**Ember:** I really believe in the importance of local art. I don't like art being perceived as this thing that only people who went to art school and have abundant surplus income can make, or this weird thing where people all over the world are consuming the same media and there's this monoculture, kind of like a flattening of local cultures. So what Shakesqueer also does is it reminds us that we are artists, and builds on and contributes to local culture.

**Sophie:** I was teaching high school when we were doing *As You Like It* and talked to a couple of my students about it, and they were like, "What? You can do Shakespeare but queer?" Just having that conversation with young people, and being able to present different storytelling and representational things, felt huge.

**Dominique:** My friend's kid, she just turned twelve, and I was really excited for her to be in the audience for *Romeo and Juliet*. For her to see a queer love story, I think that's very beautiful in and of itself, but also for her to see how fun costumes can be, and how there's this world of theater that exists where you can yell and stomp and fall to the ground and cry and have a choreographed fight sequence. You can be whoever you are, be this other character, this badass, this very vulnerable person.

**Inmn:** Theater is a real-life experience. You have to leave your house to see a play and be there with the actors. If the actors put on a play, and part of the play moves, maybe the audience moves with the play, maybe the play roves, and maybe they go do some other stuff and it becomes unclear whether it's part of the performance or whether it's a political action in and of itself.

I grew up watching Bread and Puppet and the Beehive Collective put on performances that were connected to political struggles going on.[6] I've always really loved how theater is something for the people, less so than the ruling class. Theater traditionally has been this fun way that class hierarchies can be temporarily broken down. You can get away with a lot that you couldn't normally get away with and poke a lot of fun at the ruling class in ways that at least historically,

---

6. For more on these projects, see Bread and Puppet, https://breadandpuppet.org/; Beehive Collective, https://beehivecollective.org/.

people might have been much more heavily reprimanded for, or were killed or imprisoned for.

The theater provides this shield—I mean, it's not a thick shield; it's pretty paper thin—against repression or consequences because it is playful, although I think that is less true now than it was during the Middle Ages or Renaissance. One of the traditional pieces of Halloween was that you could go and demand food from rich people, and if they didn't give it to you, it was perfectly legal to throw rocks at their house and shit. But if people did that now, they'd probably get in a lot of trouble. So when I think about what Shakesqueer could do as far as that in our current time and context, I think about things like that, about how we can draw attention to a lot of struggles that are going on that we're implanting into or amplifying within the plays. I would love it if in the future, we used the productions to push the envelope with current struggles a little more.

That said, queer and anarchist theater can create spaces for people to play around with ideas in physical and somatic ways that they might only ever get to think about. My hope is that by providing these temporary spaces, those moments can persist beyond the performance.

**Egg:** Theater in my experience has offered the most potential to the people who participate in it. It's an invitation to frolic in a world where the rules have changed, and that invites a reimagining of political, interpersonal, and social possibilities. Theater enables us as creators of a project to inhabit different selves, and try on how we could move these hauntings and the possession of ourselves into our everyday life.

Theater is also a space for radical possibility in that the

creation of a temporary project for the purpose of enjoyment and art and creativity invites us to step away from the pressures that a lot of us feel to be creating things for lasting glory, or padding our egos in more structured and long-term projects. In theater, instead, we are creating things together and then dismantling them, either every night or at the end of the project. The temporariness of the experience is part of what's beautiful about it. This festival-like thing.

**Adrian:** We love putting on these productions for our communities so they can see and feel the joy—or this year, mourning—of the story, but also it's for the people who are in it to have this intense feeling of putting everything aside in their life. The potential in that is that you get comfortable, and experience creating something beautiful and new, and really hard, with a group of radicals that share your vision of what the future should be. Then you get to show the whole community what you've done and the artistry, but I think honing our skills of consensus and collaboration and storytelling creates room for other projects. You could say there are parallels between doing a direct action as well. Being in a group of people where you're trying to figure something out together and collaborate, and it's uncomfortable, and you have to put everything in your life aside for it.

**Glen:** Another way of putting it would be that we're demonstrating something to ourselves by doing it. Some cool things about theater are that it's big, it makes a splash, it's an event, it's one night or three nights. I think it's important to me, from the way that I relate to art, not just to have a consumerist relationship to art, and as an artist or consumer, you have to be dodging out of it because that's the hegemonic way of relating to it. We proved to ourselves that first year that not only could we tell a story in this big way of freezing time and gathering everybody to share in this storytelling but we also felt that it was worth doing just for the sake of doing it. That way of relating to art could potentially feed into a way of relating to society in general.

**Ember:** I love the idea of touring. I was really excited when we learned that there's an anarchist theater festival in Montreal. In my dream, I was like, "We're gonna get a school bus and fill it up with our set and the band and whatever, and drive to Montreal and have the best time, the most outrageously fun time we could possibly imagine." I hope that's not impossible in the future. But it's perfectly good for Shakesqueer to stay the scale that it is, and it's important for the people who are putting it on and the people who are the audience.[7]

**Maggie:** It's been really nice with Shakespeare that we can adapt a play to touch on themes of queerness or feminism or radical politics in general. But I hope that we're giving people the skills and confidence to do storytelling through theater that's maybe even more blatantly radical. Before Shakesqueer, I didn't really know anyone doing theater in Tucson. And since Shakesqueer, a lot of our friends now have different skills around it. The more ways that we know how to tell stories, the better, because I think stories are powerful when it comes to pushing these ideas into the realm of reality.

---

7. Another group, Shakesqueer Vermont, began in 2022 with a production of *Romeo and Juliet*.

✿  ✿  ✿

Wren Awry is a Tucson-based writer, archivist, and editor of the anthology *Nourishing Resistance: Stories of Food, Protest, and Mutual Aid* (PM Press, 2023).

Shakesqueer Tucson produces radical, queer interpretations of Shakespeare plays. You can learn more about its work at www.shakesqueertheater.org.

# COMMUNITARIAN KITCHENS: STOKING THE FLAMES OF MEMORY AND REBELLION

/

VILMA ROCÍO ALMENDRA
QUIGUANÁS, TRANSLATED BY SCOTT
CAMPBELL

Our relationship with our territories is woven into the *tulpas*, the millennia-old fires of encounters, legacies, flavors, and knowledges. Memory is spun, and the fires of resistance and freedom are rekindled. Today, there are those who try to usurp this space of flames and affects, to glamorize it, and turn it into an image and propaganda so as to later steal it, empty it of meaning, and destroy it as a passing fad or merchandise. The tulpa, though, this center of women in collectivity with the land and family, this heart of liberation and intimacy, this power to be ourselves without being seen or judged so as to continue surviving, has no price and cannot fit into the market. This sketch recalls the tulpas, invokes them, and calls on us to care for ourselves by caring for them. It is the life around the fire that keeps us going.

When neighborhood women feel the same needs, when neighbors talk about their problems, or when neighbors come together and feel the same hunger, many times they self-organize around food, around the fire, around their challenges. This has happened historically, and it continues to happen to this day in large and small uprisings, mobilizations, and marches, where particularly women—and all of those who labor daily to care for life—work to provide food during social actions.

For example, during the 2021 national strike in what they call Colombia, when youths issued a call to rise up against the increased taxes and cuts to health care proposed by President Iván Duque Márquez's government, and then hundreds of thousands of people seeking social transformation joined the protests, the communitarian kitchens, sustained by fire, were an essential pillar, feeding the front lines of the uprising that exploded in the streets for more than sixty days.[1] It's not known how many communitarian kitchens were created. It's only known that whoever passed by donated what little they had in their home—rice, beans, lentils, salt, oil, potatoes, bananas, or whatever was within reach—and the various ingredients were then cooked into soups, stews, and broths in the giant communal pots that fed the mobilized masses in the cities. Groups of women and men collected the food, and then sorted and prepared it, keeping the communitarian kitchens in constant action. As people washed, peeled, chopped, seasoned, and mixed foodstuffs to create a delicious and steaming hot soup, they also shared words about the struggle in the streets, their needs, the media's lies, the repression, the resistance, and their dreams as well as life and death.

The communitarian kitchens were where youths came to enjoy a good meal and collectively fed themselves while fighting together for a common cause. In fact, some of the impoverished youths, strong on the front lines, said that during the strike, they were able to eat three times a day thanks to the communitarian kitchens. As well, families and collectives prepared food and drink in their homes, and then brought it directly to the barricades because they both wanted to take care of the mobilized youths and were indignant that the so-

---

1. *Translator's notes*: Technically, *ollas comunitarias* means "communitarian pots" in English. I've chosen to go with "communitarian kitchens" to get at the spirit of what they embody, but other translations might be "communal pots," "communal cooking pots," or "community pots," or "communal kitchens" or "community kitchens." The front lines, supported and nourished by the communitarian kitchens, were made up of women, men, and nonconforming folks who put themselves at the front of the marches, encampments, and other collective actions in order to safeguard the mobilizations and protect other people. Many of them were killed, disappeared, tortured, and/or jailed by the state.

called public forces had destroyed some of the communitarian kitchens, leaving them without food. In spite of this, the communitarian kitchens persisted in word and action during this lengthy mobilization. Hopefully they will continue to be maintained through the self-organization and solidarity of the peoples, countering any efforts to institutionalize them and make them dependent on the state.

## THE FIRE THAT INHABITS ME

Since I was a girl, fire has been an everyday part of my life. Infinite memories of our daily relationship with fire now inhabit me. The tulpas always remind me of dreams, signs, stories, advice, plants, remedies, flavors, colors, smells, and sounds. I remember the tulpa in our house in the mountains of the Indigenous reservation of Jambaló, in the southwest of what they call Colombia; its three big rocks were on the ground, almost in the center of our kitchen, with pieces of burning wood atop the stones. Always nearby were the pots of food, medicinal waters, brewed coffee, and toasted coca that provided all the energy for the day's work.

I remember my maternal grandparents, with whom I had the privilege of spending my childhood. They were always close to the tulpa, asking us about our dreams; explaining the meaning of signs (bodily vibrations) to us so that we could recognize the messages of Mother Earth; showing us how to use plants to protect ourselves and care for the territory; and advising us, based on their joys and sorrows, on how to walk through life.

They taught us how to understand the fire's signals. When the sounds of the fire seemed smothered, for instance, as if someone was blowing on the flames from inside the fireplace, it was because a visitor would arrive soon. We were then supposed to take a little bit of ash and throw it into the fire, saying aloud, "May they not come empty-handed. May they bring something." Or when the fire sparked and emitted small, sharp explosions, it meant that an ill-tempered person was going to arrive. That is what I learned from my grandmother, and that is how I live today, here and now, with my family in the mountains I inhabit.

In 2013, when I was participating in the "Little School of Freedom according to the Zapatistas" and staying in the home of a family from the bases of support, the fire there began to spark. My compañera host listened to the memories of my grandmother while we did the domestic work necessary to then eat some delicious tortillas. I explained to my compañera that an ill-tempered person was probably about to arrive. A short time later, a woman came to the house. The surprised compañera told me, "Here comes my *comadre* [friend], and yes, she is very harsh!!!"

Our relationship with fire is fundamental for familial intimacy and also territorial collectivity. The fires of familial intimacy are woven into territorial collectivity, not just due to the material support each family brings, but because of the spiritual energy that each family provides for the community. This fabric of fires has given birth to collective words and actions to defend life too, beyond the rural and urban—the locations that the state has assigned to us.

## THE COMMUNITARIAN KITCHENS

Today I relive the memory of the communitarian kitchens that we helped to stoke in the mountains of Jambaló in 1986, when my mother became a teacher in the rural community of El Voladero. Festivals and school ceremonies were held that wove us toward a better education. I remember the comadres, midwives, and neighborhood women arriving with something from their garden and a knife in hand to cook. I remember the day laborers, musicians, and neighbors arriving with firewood, and in case more was needed, machetes in hand. We held a *minga*—ancestral collective work where everyone contributes—to enjoy life in community.

We all took collective action to build a decent school, better education, happy childhood, and organized community. From that space, we dreamed and created daily life around the fire. At that time, almost everyone had a tulpa in their home. The school meetings were places to not only to talk about the progress and setbacks of the students but above all address the problems of the community and look for collective solutions. Not everything was rosy, but keeping the fire burning during the various collective actions ensured that community organization was maintained at the time.

The communitarian kitchens, better known as *fogones* in our territories, have always accompanied the communal work carried out through the mingas. They have been present in the barter exchanges and assemblies, nourished the traditional festivals, and never been absent from the mobilizations and collective actions that we have carried out for the past fifty-three years organized by the Cauca Indigenous Regional

Council in the Mother of the Forests (Kauka, in the Namtrick language of my Misak people).[2]

Our fogones have been fed by the determination and solidarities in the mountains, reciprocity between us and the land, and need to achieve a common objective among *pueblos originarios* [first or original peoples]: to recover the land. Toward this objective, my grandfather told me that they used to have big parties to gather resources, but that the police almost always arrived to tear down the communitarian kitchens and dump out the pots of chicha, a fermented maize drink, in order to hinder collective action.

Knocking down the communitarian kitchens has practically become the law. The state and police have done it everywhere so as to destabilize our organizing. Even so, the communitarian kitchens have been the heart of our territorial struggles, and with greater need in the cities now, they have become a refuge that mitigates the hunger caused by the extractivism and dispossession that commodifies the land and life itself.

In the cities, there are beautiful experiences too. There are those who have resisted the systemic crises that fall on their shoulders, thanks to the collectivity found around the fire, and have managed to feed themselves despite the impoverishment they have been subjected to in urban spaces. The coming together of those who are displaced and impoverished in the cities has allowed people to not only fight for food through the communitarian kitchens but also feed the rebellions for a dignified life.

---

2. The council was created in 1971 to fight for the unity, land, culture, and autonomy of the peoples in the mountains of the Cauca.

## FIRE FEEDS THE BODY AND SPIRIT

In the uprisings, strikes, revolts, marches, encampments, popular assemblies, blockades, land recuperations, communal congresses, appropriation of factories, roadblocks, and popular tribunals, and on pickets and barricades, fire has always been present.

Fire helps us to endure low temperatures and cook food so as to resist, among many other things. Communitarian kitchens and fire are a necessary couple. They have been present and vital in feeding the dignified rebellions that denounce and question the state, transnationals, and all the other powers that have always oppressed us. For the most part, the communitarian kitchens have been the fruit of self-organization, self-management, and self-care, far beyond the promises and lies of the state.

For a long time, in ruralized and urbanized territories, communitarian kitchens have sustained struggles against hunger, for land and water, as a life practice and central axis for collective nourishment. Without going too far back, it is enough to recall some exemplary moments in various latitudes that have stoked the fires of struggle.

There is the Housewives Committee of the Twentieth-Century Mine founded in the 1960s by the wives of tin miners at the Siglo XX Mine in Potosí in what they call Bolivia. These women organized against the repression and imprisonment of their husbands, who had marched for the payment of wages. They demanded the miners' freedom, food supplies, and payment for work. Among them, Domitila Barrios de Chungara distinguished herself as one of the most courageous.

Then too, there is the Villa El Salvador Self-Managed Urban Community, which arose in 1973 from the efforts of impoverished families in Lima in what they call Peru, where women organized themselves to guarantee food. In this context, María Elena Moyano, one of the great examples of this self-managed community, founded the Micaela Bastidas Mothers' Club, concerned with women's issues, education, and family health.

Also, in Veracruz in the place they call Mexico, there is the inspiration of Leonila Vásquez, who in 1994, moved by the Central American migrants passing through on the "Bestia" (train of death) to reach their "American dream," decided to share what little she had for her family and deliver it via "launches," throwing bags of food onto the train for the migrants. Today there are more women, known as the Protectors, who continue Leonila's legacy and now have more support to carry out this humanitarian work.

And there is the *piqueteros* (picketers) movement, born at the end of the 1990s in Buenos Aires in the place they call Argentina. "Pickets" (roadblocks and blockades) were erected in various parts of the city in rejection of the precariousness of work and resultant hunger caused by rampant neoliberalism. In 2001, the pickets grew stronger, along with the bravery and dignity of the women—visible because they were not only a fundamental part of the communal feeding but in all areas of care during the pickets as well.

This is just a sample of an endless number of illustrations. Yet without a doubt, the eighty bonfires of Cherán in the Purépecha Plateau of what they call Mexico are our reference point. Day and night for more than six months in 2011, the people of Cherán resisted, ignited by women setting bonfires, which in turn became the spark for the *K'eri* communal self-governance there that today inspires and infects the world.[3]

During the pandemic, hunger, discontent, and indignation were what compelled people to organize. People clearly saw the need to collectively feed themselves in order to resist economic subjugation, urgency to rise up together in the face of policies and reforms that continue to impoverish them, and necessity to decide how to sustain the various uprisings and safeguard life. Moreover, against the backdrop of rising fascism, social abandonment, and the current wars and others in the making, it is not enough to name the self-proclaimed Front Line Mothers of the communitarian kitchens in what they call Chile or Ecuador, Colombia or Peru—the women who are fundamental to self-managing everything in daily life, and more so when they come together and manage to feed revolutions. We must also mention the mothers, women, children, and youths who day by day are being bombed, displaced, and disappeared, and impeded from having their own communitarian kitchens.

## TO INHABIT OBSCURITY AND CARE FOR THE TULPAS

There are many other communitarian kitchens that don't declare themselves as such. They, made up mostly of women, simply provide dignified food for the resistances and feeling-thinking that walk side by side during concrete actions. That is, from what we've witnessed recently in the resistances in

---

3. For the story of these bonfires and the communal self-governance structures that arose from them, see Scott Campbell, "The Bonfires of Autonomy in Cherán," in *Deciding for Ourselves: The Promise of Direct Democracy*, ed. Cindy Milstein (Chico, CA: AK Press, 2020), 161–98.

Abya Yala [the Americas], it is not enough to list the self-managed spaces, write down the names of communitarian kitchens, and quote the words of the women cooking to enumerate the fullness of collective actions.

We must go beyond the spotlight. We must gather ourselves in the shadows to ensure that communitarian kitchens come together through self-organization, self-care, and self-management, and don't get lost in welfare politics that try to bureaucratize even food. May they not get lost in the institutionalization that political parties seek. May they not turn into banners for the compañera or compañero from the struggle who transforms themselves into a candidate in order to take power from above. May they continue to germinate as seeds that bloom in soil fertilized by dignified rebellion and the urgency of autonomy.

In a context where the powers from above have shown us that no matter how libertarian they may be, they must always comply with the regime of sacrificing the people (it's enough to look into the mirror at Venezuela, Nicaragua, Chile, and Bolivia), our fires are crucial. In a context where other pandemics such as hunger are looming, wars continue to be the biggest business, extractivism continues to triumph, patriarchy continues to turn the land into merchandise, the communitarian kitchens are an emergent necessity to sustain life and collective relations among peoples. This continues to be demonstrated here and now by the Network of Community Kitchens in Popayán. I invite us to immerse ourselves in the obscurity that inhabits the *ollas comunitarias* when the lights of the spectacle cease to shine on the sweaty faces and calloused hands behind the steaming pots.

※ ※ ※

Vilma Rocío Almendra Quiguanás, daughter of the Nasa and Misak peoples, is a member of Pueblos en Camino (pueblosencamino.org), a self-managed initiative that seeks to weave resistance and autonomy among peoples and processes in Abya Yala. She can be contacted at https://facebook.com/almendra.kiwenasa or vilmaalmendra@yahoo.es. Vilma resides in Vereda Quitapereza, Santander de Quilichao, Mother of the Forests, in what they call Colombia.

Scott Campbell is a radical writer and translator residing in both what they call the United States and Mexico. His personal website is fallingintoincandescence.com. He'd like to thank Anthony Dest and Valeria Peña for their assistance on this project.

# SUPPORTING THE REVOLUTION, ONE STEW AT A TIME

/

ALEH STANKOVA AND
FENYA FISCHLER

Growing up in a Balkan household, without the excess of capitalist-driven consumption (in the 1990s at least), I (Aleh) was used to collective ownership, hand-me-downs, knowing aunties and uncles you could get in touch with if you wanted to get this or that done, and sharing and taking care of the resources you had because no one could afford replacements. Later on, it was through Food Not Bombs that I really grew to appreciate mutual aid networks and care for one another in a deliberate way, though. Indeed, many of us in the North London Food Not Bombs chapter embodied queer, femme, and migrant identities. We were also looking for a community where we could share our true selves with one another and put our politics into practice, beyond waged labor relationships and exploitation, beyond the imperialist and racist attitudes of white English culture, beyond the alienation and forced segregation of the rapidly gentrifying mega city of London.

We first met in around 2010 in Colchester, a small town in Essex in the United Kingdom, where we were both studying at the time. Our first conversation happened over a pot of simmering stew that was later carried outdoors for a food share. From there, we shared many conversations around anarchism, mutual aid, feminist politics, and practice, and as our friendship solidified and grew stronger, so did our politics. We found that exploring our lives and organizing through an anarcha-feminist lens told us a lot about our own experiences, what we wanted our friendship to look like, and what we wanted our community and political projects to reflect. So a couple years later, when we decided to establish a Food Not Bombs chapter in London with a small group of friends, it seemed natural and essential that the values that had guided us and sustained our relationships would be at the core of any initiative we cocreated.

Our first-ever cooking session together was at the first AFem conference in London in 2014. We showed up sleep deprived to the communal kitchen and cooked a giant pot of warm food, which we then carried by hand to the anarcha-feminist conference venue. We set up a simple table with our pots in the center of a hallway, and a queue started forming soon after. And we stayed there until every portion of food had been served and we had a clear view of the bottom of the pot again. As we shared food, we spoke to people who said they hadn't been able to afford to eat all day and this was their first warm meal in days. Having access to free, tasty food gave them the energy they needed to take part in the discussions and workshops. This experience really drove home the point that we can't separate our political selves from our bodies.

Since then, as the two longest-running members, we saw our Food Not Bombs chapter shift across various London neighborhoods between 2014 and 2021, but we also found a place to call home: our collective. We did that on the solid ground of those who came before us. In fact, one of our most prized items was passed down to us through a person living in Angel (an area of London) who got in touch to say that he'd hung onto a sturdy old pot used by his now-defunct Food Not Bombs. Could we please make use of it? It still had the group's initials in marker on the side and an old piece of string left on one of the handles many eons ago.

For years we lugged that sixty-liter steel cooking pot around on bicycles, in all sorts of baggage compartments, on public transport, by hand, in pairs and fours, with hot stews fogging people's glasses as they waddled over to wherever we'd set up our stall that time. This pot ended up feeding the neighbors, feminists, migrants, houseless folks, people using drugs, sex workers, families, students, and friends who would come to our stall to share a hot meal, cup of tea, and whatever useful items we'd scrounged that week—from menstrual pads to sleeping bags, dog food or crates of veggies, or antimilitarist and anticapitalist literature. To do that, we'd actively reach out to neighborhood businesses for their leftover food, trek with big backpacks at 5:00 a.m. to wholesale markets halfway across the city, or in the early days when supermarket bins weren't behind big walls and lock and key, go dumpster diving. All of this allowed us to consistently be at a corner twice a month, including when we found our most permanent spot, Seven Sisters station in the borough of Haringey, where we shared food and know-your-rights literature at a joint stall with the local group resisting immigration raids.

The planning, coordination, and physical labor required to cook a meal for dozens of people was a humbling and beautiful experience for all who took part. Often we started the day exhausted after a long week of wage labor, but left energized by the community spirit and commitment of everyone who was able to take part. Caring for others felt like caring for ourselves too. We're told repeatedly that the answer to our burnout or tiredness is to just rest and even withdraw from organizing—which is of course sometimes necessary. But we don't acknowledge enough how solidarity, collective care, and direct action can also provide us with essential ingredients to boost our spirits and keep us going: hope, joy, togetherness, support, friendship, and more.

We balanced many responsibilities, including full-time (or more) jobs, with sustaining our chapter of Food Not Bombs. As part of this work, we tried (sometimes definitely more successfully than at other moments) to challenge capitalist ways of working that push us beyond our limits so that we can "achieve." We did our best to be honest about our energy in a world that forces us to separate ourselves from the needs of our bodies, and we didn't pressure ourselves to "push through" if there wasn't enough capacity to make something happen. We supported each other in taking breaks as well as in making sure the work was joyful, loving, and revolved around connection and relationships with each other. For us, it was crucial to maintain a space that felt nourishing in many ways, not only physically, but emotionally.

The relationships we formed through our organizing were a big part of what allowed us to sustain this group for so long (to our knowledge, we're the longest-running Food Not Bombs chapter to have ever existed in London!). Centering relationships also meant being clear about the types of networks we wanted to build: reciprocal, horizontal, caring, and supportive. We truly believe that our group survived despite the odds because of the intentionality with which we built up our political practice, aligning with feminist and anarchist values that saw us resisting engrained hierarchies and patriarchal organizing patterns, and how that manifested in the way we looked out for each other.

Being in a public space as mostly women, femmes, and queers, we unfortunately did face occasional sexism and patronizing comments. When members were confronted with sexual harassment at our stalls, we would intervene to protect each other and make it clear that such behavior wasn't acceptable at our food shares. One time we dealt with a man who seriously insisted that we serve him with our "lady hands," which we refused with humor, but not without frustration. In another instance, once when we returned to one of our kitchen spots in a local community center, we found that our IWW poster, aimed at men and boys with the phrase "The Revolution Begins in the Sink!," had been defaced by a man who seemed to have taken offense at it.

While we worked in a horizontal way through consensus, we were aware that many groups without formal hierarchies in practice end up reproducing informal power dynamics that remain unacknowledged. Rather than pretending they didn't exist, we made time, when we could, to reflect on and acknowledge those dynamics among ourselves. Moreover, we tried to figure out how we could pass on, instead of centralize, knowledge and connections, better encourage others in our group to take up space, and build a kitchen that felt welcoming and inclusive, where questions were welcomed as well. This happened through regular meetings along with informal and annual strategy days where everyone could speak freely about group dynamics and newer members could take ownership of where we were heading as a collective. For a lot of us, this type of open communication and space to challenge and subvert hidden hierarchies within collectives had been sorely missing in organizing spaces we'd been part of previously (and even now). We've seen a lot of those other spaces fall apart because there is resistance to centering this type of caring accountability as an organizing practice.

Our Food Not Bombs experience left us with the conviction

that relationships and care labor are absolutely essential to movements and organizing. Direct action and political interventions aren't just about marching down streets with the black bloc, picketing racist and exploitative employers, and puncturing police and immigration vans' tires—and if that's what they look like, they can and should take place on a full belly! In short, care (including food), which is so often devalued and gendered, is in fact the invisible fuel that sustains us in the struggle. Emphasizing only the most visible, frontline, or confrontational forms of activism fails to acknowledge the massive amounts of labor carried out every day that may look quite different, but are still part of the glue that holds us all together. It also creates a harmful standard, the socially accepted figure of the "activist," against which only able-bodied folks and those who don't face disproportionate risks due to their immigration status, race, ethnicity, or gender identity and expression can measure up to.

Over the years we swung ladles in the kitchen for and with prison abolitionists, antiwar demonstrations, sex workers' conferences, migrant rights groups, feminist meetings on intimate partner violence, and many more. None of us were professional cooks, except for the few times someone with that background happened to join in. We tried to be both pragmatic and creative, and figure out simple recipes based on the various vegetables and staple foods we had available at any given time. Sometimes, shut away in kitchens while others labored on strategies and organizing techniques, we worried about whether we would be perceived as reproducing the same patriarchal, gendered dynamics that historically and disproportionately put femme people there. Yet that was quickly dispelled during shared chats and meals. Once, for instance, we cooked in a community center for a collective providing support to arrestees. We barely saw their faces the whole time. Warm, nutritious food awaited them when they took a break from what turned out to be a challenging and complex discussion about their future work. They told us later that being cooked for in this way throughout the day made them feel cared for and supported so as to stay grounded and wade through difficult conversations together.

Whenever we cooked for organizers, picket lines, protests, and different collectives, we brought with us this understanding: sharing food publicly, for free and to whomever shows up, was an unexpectedly subversive act in a world where we are always expected to earn a living and earn our survival, where we have to prove we're deserving of compassion and care, or repent before being deemed worthy of basic necessities. We actively challenged the few people who treated us like a catering service and expected to be served and waited on like they were in a restaurant. Based on our experiences, we developed written guidelines setting out our ways of working, including that we were not service providers. We made it clear that we opposed classist, patronizing, and tokenistic attitudes internalized by passersby who felt that the food we shared should only have been given to "people in need" or "the homeless." We refused to engage in the capitalist power dynamics of top-down humanitarian work that divides people into service providers and service users. We practiced solidarity, not charity.

This meant that we would not accept gatekeeping in our cooking and food-sharing spaces. In a gentrified, expensive city where barely anyone can afford to own a home or car, or have the room required to cook a big meal, we were always on the lookout for the next kitchen and storage space we could use as a base. Over the years we had many spots—kitchens in our homes, homeless shelters, or community centers, with pots and pans, grains and canned goods, stacked on each other in our living rooms and people's sheds.

Over those same years, we were also a political home for many people—those just arriving in London would look us up, and we hosted many visitors who joined us for a cooking session while they were on the rainy island we called home for a while. Whenever I (Fenya) would travel, I'd do the same: look up the local Food Not Bombs chapter and join it for a food-sharing session. From sharing food on the streets of Tijuana, to distributing dozens of burritos from the trunk of a car in Skid Row, to militant picnics during antiwar protests in London, I immediately felt at home chopping veggies and figuring out how to support the revolution one stew at a time.

❊ ❊ ❊

Aleh Stankova is a queer Balkan feminist organizer originally from Bulgaria who spent many years living in the United Kingdom, where she cofounded North London Food Not Bombs. She is currently based in Sofia, Bulgaria. Aleh has worked extensively within feminist and women's rights organizations, including with victims of domestic and state violence, and by resourcing feminist movements. She is also trying to DJ, and is an auntie and proud cat parent.

Fenya Fischler is currently based in Brussels, where she's involved in diasporist and queer Jewish organizing. Prior to moving to Belgium, she spent most of her adult life living in the United Kingdom, where she cofounded and organized with North London Food Not Bombs. She has been working for over a decade to support feminist, queer, and other movements globally. When she's not organizing, Fenya enjoys hanging out with her cats, studying Yiddish, and singing.

You can find the North London Food Not Bombs group on Instagram @fnb_london and Facebook @fnblondon.

# AN EXPERIMENT
# IN ADDRESSING
# INTRAORGANIZATIONAL
# VIOLENCE

/

BENJI HART

What would it actually take to end sexual violence in grassroots social movements? How do we dismantle massive and entrenched institutions while simultaneously confronting the ways that we as individuals have internalized those institutions' harmful practices? If our movements are only as strong as our communities, how do we build up both in ways that are committed to fighting gender-based violence for the long haul? How do we make concrete commitments to collective care with the understanding that the apparatuses of the state—including war and militarism—are themselves a source of sexual violence and not the answer to it?

These were some of the key questions I asked alongside a small group of organizers as we attempted to plot out the policies and procedures around addressing sexual violence for a new configuration, Dissenters. We did so with the intent of imagining new structures to hold our movements—ones created through a feminist anarchist lens—that centered the needs of the most marginalized members of our communities and made fighting sexual violence a high priority instead of an afterthought.

A youth antiwar organization, Dissenters was launched in 2020 in Chicago, Illinois, only months before the COVID-19 lockdown and subsequent George Floyd uprisings. The goal of the new formation was to reenergize Black and Brown youth-led efforts to combat war profiteers, weapons manufacturers, and Western imperialism globally. It also aspired to reclaim the antiwar movement from much of its white liberal leadership and toothless calls for "peace," which often fail to connect US militarism abroad to its insidious iterations in Black, Indigenous, and migrant communities in the United States itself.

Dissenters' cofounders worked diligently for months leading up to the launch and remotely throughout the pandemic. They tweaked the organization's chapter-based model, which looks to college campuses as an initial locus for antiwar agitation, and defined its vision, core principles, and internal structures, all with the aim of creating an organization that could withstand attacks from the behemoth military-industrial complex as well as the internal conflicts that regularly take our projects down from the inside.[1] It was from this latter place that the cofounders identified the dire need to address sexual violence within the organization before it got off the ground.

As one of the original members of the Safety through Practice and Accountability (SPA) team—the internal mechanism meant to both build a culture of consent within Dissenters from the beginning and provide resources and support in anticipation of potential intraorganizational violence—I joined a crew that included many people who themselves are survivors of gender, partner, and sexual violence within radical spaces. We had each been, if not the direct recipients of harm, then witnesses to the ways that interpersonal violence and its mismanagement can destroy the relationships necessary to maintain movements along with the communities that comprise them. The tired responses of shielding individuals from accountability due to their social importance, and treating the addressing of sexual violence as secondary to "real" organizing, were recurring attitudes that had undermined or even ended previous efforts we'd been part of.

---

1. For more information on Dissenters, see wearedissenters.org.

These experiences motivated our initial work with Dissenters' SPA team—not merely wanting to avoid the pitfalls that had wrecked other attempts, but understanding that ending war is impossible without ending sexual violence. Any antiwar effort led by youths, women, and trans and queer people cannot separate militarism from the specific ways that war relies on gender-based violence to target those same groups. As individuals who belong to those identities, prioritizing resistance to intercommunal harm in the antiwar movement is also about centering our own protection in the struggle to end state repression. Acknowledging the shortfalls of our previous efforts—and our own imperfectness as organizers—we wanted to shape new spaces where fighting sexual violence and defending its targets was a core commitment, and where sharpening our tools to do so was a collective practice.

As our inaugural contribution to Dissenters, we designed a member handbook, or more of a zine, to be widely shared throughout the organization. The handbook strived to clearly outline the organization's policies and best practices surrounding consent and sexual violence, connect the work of resisting gender-based violence back to the primary principles of antiwar organizing, and recruit every member at every level of the organization to commit to that work. Some key themes emerged as we performed the complicated labor of trying to imagine the very structures that we ourselves had never actually seen, and that might have stopped previous campaigns we'd been a part of from going off the rails.

## WE ARE ALL OF US AND NONE OF US EXPERTS

Even coming up with the name for our team took some trial and error. We ultimately landed on Safety through Practice and Accountability because we wanted to make two things clear to the larger organization. For one, we are not experts, because if any one individual had figured out how to end sexual violence, our movements would have already eliminated it. And second, we are not here to provide easy answers but rather to offer resources, structures, and intentional spaces for all members of the organization to practice flexing their own muscles in responding to sexual harm, and building chapters where a commitment to fighting gender-based violence is woven into every action and conversation.

Our aim here was to both set realistic expectations and make our intentions explicit from the onset. When those from marginalized identities experience violence in our own spaces, there can be a deep disappointment layered on top of the trauma, as we frequently arrived at those spaces because we were fleeing the violence of others—our families, our jobs, our schools, and larger institutions. We can understandably have higher expectations for how we will be treated in spaces that are explicitly feminist, antiracist, and antiauthoritarian, by their very nature promising us a vision of a better world. When we experience the same harm there that we did in the spaces we escaped, the feeling of betrayal can amplify the pain of the harm itself.

What the handbook attempts to communicate is not, "You will never experience harm here," but instead, "If and when harm likely does happen, here are the ways we are collectively committing to responding to it." We aren't promising to have answers or get it right every time; we're promising to practice together, give our best efforts, reflect when we get it wrong, and be accountable to one another in the process. The SPA team is not a police force poised to punish those who break our policies; it is a support system meant to infuse better practices of accountability throughout the organization. To this end, the handbook even includes a flowchart that members can follow to determine whether a conflict or miscommunication requires them to reach out to the SPA team, or if there are already methods and resources at their disposal to help them address it on their own.

We hope this honest framing will help to avoid future letdowns and disillusionment, while demonstrating that we are dedicated to thinking through our responses to gender-based and sexual violence from the jump, not merely after violence occurs. We also hope this will make explicit that while none of us as individuals have all the answers, collectively we have hundreds of experiences of preventing, resisting, and healing from violence that are the true fodder to help us build out new structures. We trust this will facilitate a shift away from looking to a core of "experts" who must answer all of our questions and solve our problems for us, to our movements assuming collective responsibility for the fighting of gender-based violence, to diving into the messy work and becoming more expert as we experiment together.

❖   ❖   ❖

## BOUNDARIES ARE NOT BORDERS

Dissenters coach Dylan Rodriguez, an author and scholar, teaches us that "a boundary is not a border."[2] A theme we noticed in organizing spaces—particularly those involving youths—is that a commitment to tearing down oppressive structures can sometimes unintentionally result in the erosion of norms and expectations that are crucial to reinforcing relationships of trust.

An example of this might be a group declaring, in a genuine attempt to fight adultism, that adults and young people are completely equal within the organization. While this might seem just and even radical at the onset, it can often lead to dynamics where the real social power that adults have over youths is denied, making it easier for older members to manipulate and pressure young people into unhealthy or even violent relationship dynamics. Much like the insistence on not "seeing" race, denying the existence of racism, ableism, sexism, and other forms of systemic violence doesn't make them go away but rather frequently allows them to flourish.

As the SPA team, one of our guiding beliefs is that borders control us, but boundaries protect us. Anarchist feminist politics do not teach us to reject all structure. They invite us to imagine structures that are shaped by and intended to protect the autonomy of the most vulnerable versus the interests of the most powerful.

To avoid these dynamics and embody these aspirations, we

---

2. Dylan Rodriguez, Dissenters Safety Protocol Training for Coaches, October 27, 2021. For an introduction to Rodriguez and his work, see https://profiles.ucr.edu/app/home/profile/dylanr.

came up with some hard-and-fast rules. The handbook makes it specifically clear that adult members of the organization are prohibited from entering into romantic or sexual relationships with Dissenters students. But it also attempts to stay dynamic and grapple with gray areas; for instance, it doesn't ban or discourage any substance use but instead offers honest reflections on the ways substances inherently complicate consent, and tips for avoiding inappropriate behavior when altered. There's even a section with specific tools for communicating boundaries and responding with reflection in place of defensiveness when someone communicates a boundary to us.

## DESTIGMATIZING THE OWNING OF HARM, WHILE NOT NORMALIZING HARM ITSELF

Another of our movement mentors, grassroots organizer and author Mariame Kaba, reminds us that you cannot actually hold anyone accountable.[3] We set ourselves up for all types of futile power struggles as well as deep heartbreak when we enter the work of transformative justice with this expectation. Within the handbook, we talked about how it is on each of us as individuals to hold ourselves accountable when another member of our collective comes to us and expresses we've done something that hurt them. What the collective can do is to help foster the conditions and create the containers within which individuals who have caused harm—which will likely be every one of us eventually—can willingly take responsibility for the consequences of their actions.

We tried to offer a framework for this in our handbook,

---

3. "Why Is This Happening? Thinking about How to Abolish Prisons with Mariame Kaba" (podcast), April 10, 2019.

starting with the notion that if we accept that sexual violence is pervasive because we are all shaped by and participating in various ways in a culture that allows its proliferation, then the confrontation of gender-based violence requires that we all change everyday aspects of how we interact with one another. Many who have experienced violence in radical spaces can attest that the initial harm is often only part of the damage that caused them to walk away from organizations and campaigns. It is equally the individual who caused the harm's inability to own what they did and acknowledge how hurtful their actions were—or even that the harm happened. What can hurt even more is the community leaping to defend harm doers in ways that they were unwilling or unable to defend the person who was exposed to the harm in the first place.

So much of changing this internal culture is actually not about promising perfect communities—something we make sure not to do in the handbook. Even under the most ideal conditions and with our best intentions, we will continue to mess up, miscommunicate, and hurt each other. Rather, the goal is to change the ways we respond when violence takes place. If we want people to own their harmful behavior, we have to be willing to create spaces for them to do so, and not merely push them out of community when they make a mistake. If we want others to believe in our capacity to change our own behavior, to hold ourselves to account when we have caused harm, we have to be willing to do the same for others.

This puts us in a tricky position, which we tried hard to wrestle with in the handbook. On the one hand, we are sincere when we say we want to end sexual violence in our spaces. On the other hand, we can only achieve this if we successfully foster a culture in which the knee-jerk reaction of those accused of violence isn't defensiveness and denial. We are, in other words, charged with both destigmatizing the act of coming forward and owning up to harm while not trivializing the harm itself.

Acknowledging the ubiquitousness of gender-based violence means recognizing that it has nothing to do with "good" and "bad" people, "perpetrators" and "victims." It is about a culture of violence in which we are all actively participating. We must own our role in perpetuating cycles if we are serious about stopping them. In doing so, we have to model taking responsibility for harmful behavior, removing as much of the fear of owning up to violence as possible, without falling into the trap of minimizing the violence itself. This complicated task is a gift to our future selves, as we should all expect to be in the position of taking responsibility for hurt we've caused at some point. It is about both refocusing on rooting out the harm while alleviating the shame of taking responsibility for that harm, reframing accountability as a form of healing as much for the harm doer as the recipient.

## THE HEART OF THE EXPERIMENT

As members of the SPA team, we initially presented our handbook and some of the philosophies and guidelines outlined here at Dissenters' first in-person convening since the start of the pandemic, the Tidal Wave Convergence in September 2022, with over sixty member-leaders from across our chapters and campaigns in attendance. The reception was earnest, warm, and even exciting. Many of the students and youths present expressed that they had never had frank conversations about sexual violence in an organizing space before, and were grateful for Dissenters' intentional acknowledgment of the subject and transparent approach to its procedures.

We tried to stress the same thing to them that I hope to emphasize here: this is an experiment. Like all experiments, there's a chance it won't work. We should expect that some of these policies and practices may result in real victories in terms of changing our internal movement culture, while others may fall flat or even lead to the exact same dynamics we set out to eliminate. It was great to get so much positive feedback on a document that was years in the making, especially on procedures that we ourselves spent months critiquing, redrafting, and troubleshooting. Yet as much as we have attempted to be proactive, our best planning may be for naught when we are actually faced with real instances of sexual violence within Dissenters—the likelihood of which has been diminished due to the sheer newness of the organization and the pandemic's demand for remote organizing.

But even in uncertainty, we continue forward with one final core reflection: more than any policy or procedure, it is our social relationships that determine our sense of security. Whereas the state tells us that it is strangers who mean us harm, and police, militaries, prisons, and borders that will protect us, we know that in actuality, both violence and safety are much more likely to originate with those closest to us. It is the nature of our relationships and the commitments we actively foster therein that either maintain cultures of harm or generate structures of safety.

Ultimately, this handbook and the team that created it

are meant to help the organization foster strong, interwoven relationships predicated on fighting gender-based violence, practicing stronger communication, respecting each other's boundaries, and recognizing and taking responsibility for harm when it inevitably occurs, all while simultaneously training up and supporting fierce, effective antimilitarist campaigners and organizers. Though it may be an experiment, we see it—like the handbook itself—as more than a mere attempt at shifting behavior. Our zine—and the practices it hopefully cultivates— is a love letter to our people, our collective struggles, and a world free from sexual violence that we believe is on its way.

❖ ❖ ❖

Benji Hart is an interdisciplinary author, artist, and educator whose work centers Black radicalism, queer liberation, and prison abolition. Their words have appeared in numerous anthologies, and been published at the *Advocate*, *Teen Vogue*, *Time*, and elsewhere. They have led popular education and arts-based workshops for organizations internationally, in- cluding the American Repertory Theater, Liberation Library, and Young Chicago Authors. For more of their work, see at BenjiHart.com. Special thanks to the other members of the SPA Team at the time of this essay's writing: Yuni Chang, Nadine Darwish, Debbie Southorn, and the mentorship of Rachel Caidor at the Help Desk.

# COLLECTIVELY FUNDING ABORTION

/

BAYLA (AKA BAY) OSTRACH

It's July 22, 2002, in Eugene, Oregon. The busy traffic flowing down the wide one-way stretch of West Eleventh Boulevard near the University of Oregon campus was accustomed to seeing protesters on the sidewalk outside the abortion clinic on Wednesdays, but this crowd was different. Even the usual antiabortion zealots arriving with their tired misogynist signs were caught off guard when they found clinic employees out front, picketing the clinic, rather than inside debriefing patients who'd just walked past the Far-Right gauntlet. Today, however, we were decrying the abrupt closure of the city's only independent abortion clinic, loss of our jobs as its employees, and lack of notice to our patients, some of whom had appointments that day.

Long home to an organization called the Federation of Feminist Women's Health Centers, Eugene had also hosted one of the federation's member clinics since 1991—an explicitly feminist abortion clinic where lay health workers were collectively charged with coordinating all care. We made decisions largely by consensus, and treated the rotating physicians as hired techs with no greater inherent power or status than a front desk person or pregnancy options counselor.[1] Yet now this clinic had suddenly closed, just the day before, with no advance warning to us—the workers—or our patients. Along with a small cluster of loyal volunteers, we'd been called into the area where staff meetings were held and peremptorily advised the clinic was closing, effective immediately; we were told to get our checks and turn in keys.

---

1. Though the language used at the time was not inclusive, the self-avowed feminist clinics that were part of the federation, including the one mentioned here, were early sources of queer- and trans-friendly health care in the 1980s and 1990s.

Stunned, we began asking obvious questions, "What about the patients scheduled for tomorrow? One of them is almost fifteen weeks!" "What about the thirteen-year-old coming from the coast? We just figured out her transportation!" "What about the patient coming in for a follow-up because she's been bleeding for two weeks?" "Where are people supposed to go now?" The uncomfortable administrator who'd been sent to deal with us by our "sister" clinic in Portland, where leadership had become increasingly corporate, couldn't or wouldn't answer our queries, including the biggest one: "Why?"

In indignant shock, we scrambled to grab everything we could on our way out. Someone saved a binder of Federation of Feminist Women's Health Clinics archival news clippings, someone else grabbed staff and volunteer phone numbers, and another person had the presence of mind to photocopy the schedule for the rest of the week—with patients' names and phone numbers. Others thought to stash folders into their bags with key protocols for patient care. And some gathered sentimental mementos such as pieces of art given to us by past patients or keepsakes from our desks. Decades of hard-won feminist health care wisdom and knowledge was collectively salvaged in our harried exit.

Instinctively, we headed to our office-away-from-the-clinic, a nearby brewery with picnic tables where we frequently went to decompress after a long clinic day. This time, our lengthy day was just beginning. Without saying much, we pulled out clunky cell phones, and started to go down the staff and volunteer list, calling the few friends and coworkers who hadn't been there with us to be fired in person. A half hour or so later, one of us had the sudden thought, "Does X know?!" Our medical director—the person legally responsible for the quality of care and physical well-being of our patients—and also, as it happened, the county medical director, was away on vacation and so had not been present at the meeting. We scanned the contact list for her cell phone number. I called her. The torrent of surprised expletives was audible to everyone at the table on that sunny patio. Somehow that made the magnitude of what was happening even greater: the feminist abortion clinic administration, a hundred miles or so up the freeway, had shut down the only independent abortion clinic between Northern California and Portland and terminated all of its staff without consulting the medical director.

Truth be told, at the time we had been organizing a union. All the Eugene clinic staff had signed union cards, but we had yet to file them with the National Labor Relations Board, much to my chagrin. We figured this was why we were fired. Yet closing the clinic, thereby risking the health of current patients and access to abortion for the entire region, seemed a drastic tactic. In fact, we later learned the then executive director had been embezzling funds from payroll tax deductions and feared our union election would bring this to light. But given this assumption at the time, the next step seemed obvious: we'd picket.

From Tuesday afternoon to the next morning—Wednesday, normally a busy abortion clinic day with patients scheduled every thirty minutes from 7:45 a.m. to 3:30 or 4:00 p.m.— we reached out to every sympathetic soul we could think of along with every friendly news outlet, every local feminist entity, local progressives, and even the then mayor, a known supporter of abortion. We ran to a copy shop to get large card stock and then went to someone's basement to letter picket signs. We negotiated our messaging and talked about our goals, seeking to reach consensus. Obviously, we wanted to force the clinic to reopen, but were we simply asking for our jobs back, or did we want to take over the Eugene clinic? Did we want to separate from the Portland administration and run it ourselves? Big discussions were in the air.

In that first twelve hours, we coalesced into a collective; (now ex) clinic workers, volunteers, and former staff who rushed to be at our sides all organically mobilized together with shared purpose. Sure, righteous indignation was a powerful uniting force, and we were angry on behalf of ourselves and each other as we looked up how to apply for unemployment, called our union organizers, and spoke of contacting a lawyer. Yet the majority of our pooled energy revolved around people in need of abortions and other care. (The clinic had also offered gynecologic care, testing for pregnancies and sexually transmitted infections, options counseling, contraceptives, naturopathy appointments, and even sliding-scale community acupuncture.)

We became laser-focused on people in rural southern Oregon, on the South Coast, from Northern California, in the high desert as well as small, economically depressed former mill towns, working at ski resorts and rodeos, or in casinos and office buildings—all the pregnant people in all the situations we'd seen over the seven years the clinic had been open. How many of them, often already driving two, three, or four hours to reach us, could drive the two additional hours to Portland? How many of them could take another day or two off work?

Get additional childcare? Find someone to loan them a working vehicle for that much longer or pay for that much more gas money? For many of us workers and volunteers who'd just been abruptly cut off from the clinic, these weren't abstract questions; many of us had first walked in as patients, then later volunteered, and then become an employee. I will always remember one person in particular because I gave her the results of her pregnancy test on my birthday one year, assisted with her abortion, took her volunteer application when she handed it in soon after, and the day the clinic was shut down, was learning to do ultrasounds alongside her as a coworker.

We were enraged that our clinic had been pulled out from under us, but equally from our community, the region, and all the pregnant people who relied on it. So when rush-hour traffic steadily streamed by us that next morning, and the befuddled antiabortion protesters showed up to find us in *their* usual spot, what motorists and demonstrators alike saw was a united collective of experienced feminist activists ready to do whatever it took to ensure abortion access—clinic or no clinic.

We didn't stop at that morning's picket line. Facing the glaring gap in safe, high-quality abortion services for pregnant people from Northern California to Portland, our crew of suddenly disenfranchised clinic employees and volunteers continued to mobilize. First we explored what it would take to compel the clinic to reopen, including through an unemployment or wrongful termination suit against the administrators. We talked with a labor lawyer about whether the fact that our signed union cards predated when we were fired would carry any weight with the Labor Relations Board. We had grand notions of running a reopened clinic ourselves as a collective. But we quickly encountered a sobering set of barriers to this aspiration, not the least of which was that the Eugene clinic was only one location within a larger 501(c)(3) organization based in Portland. Crucially, it wasn't clear the Eugene clinic could generate enough revenue to stay open as a stand-alone site—so we pivoted to the idea of forming a grassroots abortion referral network and fund. Each of these discussions operated based on a model of consent and consensus, with everyone taking turns facilitating meetings, each person having a chance to speak and share their thoughts, and all decisions reflecting a process of respectful, collective cocreation.

At now-regular meetings in various former coworkers' homes, gatherings in backyards and basements, or on porches, we shared stories of what we'd routinely seen as the greatest needs among our patients and their support people when our clinic was open. Then we collectively identified what folks in most of Oregon and Northern California would immediately need now that our site was closed:

- Guidance on which other clinics offered safe, high-quality care, up to what gestations, at what cost, and over how many days
- Access to existing financing for transportation, lodging, childcare, and the cost of abortion procedures
- New sources of funding now that many people would have to travel farther and likely go to clinics that cost more than had our feminist one

We knew that among us, with our combined years of experience in the recently closed clinic and others, we already had a lot of this information or knew where to find it—and we were ready to take on the challenge of creating a new abortion fund for pregnant people in Oregon. Or so we thought anyway.

While we did not explicitly discuss, to my memory, a guiding political principle on which to found our sexual and reproductive health organization along with the referral network and fund that it would administer (other than feminism and what would now be called reproductive justice), the ethos and practical processes we used followed the fundamental anarchist feminist ethics of collective care and informed consent. Having ourselves lost not only a key means of income but also social connection, we channeled our frustration as well as our concern for those who would have been our patients into an unprecedented mutual aid project in the region: the Network for Reproductive Options (NRO).

At the time that the NRO and larger organizing effort that enabled it began, those of us involved explicitly envisioned and understood it as a nonhierarchical collective that facilitated practical access to safe, high-quality abortion care for and with those in need. Though few involved in the creation of the fund may have called themselves anarchists at the time, we were all committed to ideals of consensus, informed consent, feminist solidarity, and collective support for each other and the people we sought to support with referrals and funding. There were frequent, long, and late meetings filled with interminable discussions about decision-making processes. Not everyone on that first picket line stayed engaged through the first year of the formal organization. Yet our goal remained steadfast, as did our process: collective care via grassroots abortion funding and referrals, made possible by grassroots feminist organizing to replace what was taken from us and our community.

In the early years (to be honest, for about ten years), this practically speaking looked like a shared cell phone (a flip phone!) that served as the referral hotline, a binder with contact information for clinics in Portland that someone in the NRO could personally vouch for, hard-copy contact sheets for recording our callers' info, and a shared backpack that held all of this and could be handed off weekly among us— all now volunteers, though eventually the NRO had a budget and funding enough to hire paid staff. Fundraising happened through a combination of impressive major donor and grant-writing work by indomitable middle-aged cis women who remembered life before *Roe* as well as the experiences of their friends and loved ones (or themselves) who'd obtained underground abortions, and creative community events. But everyone involved discussed and agreed on what we considered deal breakers: our hard lines around funders we'd never accept money from (for example, traditional reproductive health and contraception funding sources with histories or principles uncomfortably close to eugenics).

The NRO certainly was not—and still is not—the only grassroots abortion referral and funding organization to operate on principles of collective decision-making and collective care. According to comrades still working in the field, the Frontera Fund (Texas) and the Richmond Reproductive

Freedom Project (Virginia), for instance, also operate as collectives. Yet the project has continued for nearly twenty years, with the original referral line and fund recently merging with a similar organization in Washington to result in what is now the largest independent abortion fund in the United States: the Northwest Abortion Access Fund, based in the Pacific Northwest, but serving people coming to the West Coast for abortions from all over the United States. And over that time, it has remained committed to respectful, collaborative, shared decision-making with informed consent and reproductive justice at the heart of the work.

❋ ❋ ❋

Bayla (Bay) Ostrach is an applied medical anthropologist and community-based researcher and technical assistance provider based in Southern Appalachia. Beginning in 1999 and continuing through the mid-2010s, they worked in seven independent abortion clinics in two states and two countries, and cofounded the grassroots abortion fund described in this essay. In addition to studying abortion access, reproductive health and justice, and health policy, they study and work in harm reduction, drug user health, and topics related to mutual and social support, including with Castellers in Catalunya. Bay can be found @BaylaOstrach.

# ABORTION WITHOUT BORDERS

/

MEGAN MCGEE

While those who trust in states and politicians call for legislative measures to protect reproductive freedom, a network of organizations in Europe has taken a more direct approach, effectively demonstrating feminist anarchist ethics by creating an infrastructure of communal care. Like its name makes clear, Abortion without Borders stretches across nation-state lines, bringing together the Abortion Dream Team and Kobiety W Sieci (Women on the Web) in Poland, Ciocia Basia in Germany, the Abortion Network Amsterdam and Women Help Women in the Netherlands, and the Abortion Support Network in the United Kingdom.[1]

Asia, an anarchist activist from Poland who relocated to Amsterdam to work with Women Help Women, recalls how these groups met in 2017 on the initiative of one person from the United Kingdom who saw that they were all doing similar work, but separately, and suggested they join forces. "The idea was to figure out ways to get later abortions, especially for people living in places where there was no easy access to abortion services, and spread information," says Asia.

Poland is at the heart of that effort, given that its abortion laws are among the strictest in Europe. A now-famous phone number connects people seeking abortions to the Abortion without Borders' helpline. The helpline is staffed by Kobiety W Sieci, which counsels callers on their options and connects them with other groups in the network according to their

---

1. For more information on the individual collectives, see Abortion Dream Team, https://aborcyjnydreamteam.pl/; Kobiety W Sieci, https://maszwybor.net/; Ciocia Basia, https://instagram.com/ciocia.basia.berlin/?hl=en; Abortion Network Amsterdam https://abortionnetwork.amsterdam/; Women Help Women, https://womenhelp.org/; Abortion Support Network, https://asn.org.uk/.

needs. If someone in Poland wants to travel abroad to terminate a pregnancy, for instance, counselors refer them to Ciocia Basia, a queer feminist grassroots collective in Berlin dedicated to building structures of support for people coming to that city for abortion access. Or those who prefer to opt for a pharmacological abortion at home can order the necessary pills from Women Help Women's global telehealth service.

Abortion law has a complicated history in this traditionally Roman Catholic country. With the fall of Communism in the early 1990s, the church began to push for new legislation to restrict abortion access. Since 1932, the procedure had been legal in cases of rape and threats to maternal health, with a 1956 law expanding legal justifications for abortion to include "difficult living conditions." The newly elected non-Communist government passed legislation in 1993 that disqualified social and financial factors as a justification, leaving rape or incest, threats to maternal health, and fetal impairment as the only cases in which abortion was legal. In April 2016, Polish antiabortion organizations proposed a bill to ban the procedure in all cases except where the pregnant person's life was in danger, and the following September, the Sejm (one of the houses of Poland's Parliament) passed the bill. But the next month, after tens of thousands of people raged against the proposed legislation in decentralized demonstrations collectively known as the "Czarny Protest" (Black Protest) in cities across Poland, the other house of the Polish Parliament voted to reject the law.

On October 22, 2020, however, the Constitutional Tribunal effectively banned abortion almost entirely, ruling that terminating a pregnancy because of fetal defect was unconstitutional. This sparked mass demonstrations in which over four hundred thousand people took to the streets to protest the decision and the ruling right-wing Law and Justice Party. According to an official tally from the Ministry of Health, 1,074 out of the 1,110 legal abortions performed in Poland the year before the ruling were obtained due to fetal impairment or life-threatening disease. Yet the number of legal terminations offers little indication of how many Polish people terminate a pregnancy in any given year. Tens of thousands do so annually by ordering abortion pills through the mail or traveling outside the country to undergo procedural abortions in clinics.

Because of the obstacles to obtaining the procedure legally, people in Poland have largely defaulted to these options even in cases where they have a legally recognized right to have an abortion. For example, to terminate a pregnancy that is the result of a crime, a pregnant person needs a certified letter from a public prosecutor confirming that they were raped. Such bureaucratic obstacles can make it impossible to access abortion services before one is twelve-weeks pregnant, after which abortion is prohibited under any circumstances.

The collectives participating in the Abortion without Borders network noticed an immediate increase in interest in the services they provide following the October 2020 ruling. "We could absolutely feel the impact of the decision," notes Asia. "This was really devastating, on the one hand, but on the other hand, it also brought incredible amounts of solidarity and grassroots organizing, and organizing that went beyond the grassroots. ... It really affected the whole society. Also, there were huge demonstrations and protests that were,

I would say, counterproductive to what is the hope of people in power in Poland."

"Every attempt by the right-wing and conservative Polish government (and the antichoice organizations and hierarchs of the Catholic Church supporting it) was followed by a social upsurge, which translated into increased activity by feminist and anarchist circles, but also by people who had never done anything activist before," recalls Adrianna of the Abortion Dream Team.

"The struggle definitely strengthened the feminist movement in Poland and beyond," says one member of Ciocia Basia. That wave of demos, they add, "was the first encounter with feminist demands for some, and a kind of resurrection for others," and provided "an eye-opening momentum for people not connected to feminism in any way."

Adrianna notes that the 2016 protests against the proposed abortion ban were what inspired her to focus on bodily autonomy. She comes from a small town in Poland where she says the word *abortion* was never uttered in her family. "I didn't know such a thing existed until my early twenties, and then I think I was really against abortion," she says. "Then, step by step, becoming a feminist, I had to deal with this abortion issue. I realized it was about having control over your body. It really was a long journey from being a person who was against abortion to being a person who is totally, 100 percent proabortion right now." Adrianna explains that the 2016 demonstrations "brought together a great many communities, especially feminist and queer with anarchist" ones too. At the time, however, the actions of feminist queer groups were "harshly judged" by anarchist circles. "According to some, the actions from this period were only superficial, hardly revolutionary, and the potential of the Black Protest was not used as 'something stronger' that could lead to further change. In any case, it took several years to see how strong the community really was." She says the role of the Abortion Dream Team, which increased its visibility and activities after 2016, was invaluable here. "The collective has become a reference point for many activists, but also one of the most important sources of knowledge and inspiration in Poland." Today, Adrianna is part of a group of twelve people who support the Abortion Dream Team by answering questions on social media from people seeking abortions. "In Poland, because of this abortion stigma, it's very important to just spread the news," she asserts, "to let people know they will not be punished for taking abortion pills or going outside the country to get a procedural abortion."

The Abortion Dream Team's mission is to change the narrative on abortion, destigmatizing and dispelling myths about the procedure while spreading information about self-managed abortion, which involves terminating a pregnancy with the medicines mifepristone and misoprostol and does not require medical supervision. "The abortion pills give you power," remarks Adrianna. People can contact the team, via email, Facebook Messenger, or Instagram. First, volunteers inquire if the person has taken a test to be sure they are pregnant, and affirm that they want an abortion and need pills. Abortion Dream Team volunteers then instruct them on how to order abortion pills from Women Help Women in the Netherlands and share the link to that organization's order form.

Rather than purchasing these pills, the person ordering them makes a donation of seventy-five euros (about eighty US dollars), although they can give more if they're able. "If you don't have the money, as many people under eighteen who write us don't, we can ask the organization to waive the donation," Adrianna says, adding that "for people in Poland, it's a steep amount of money. Many of the women already have kids and can't afford to donate." The pills, which take a maximum of twenty days to arrive, are discreetly packaged, with only the recipient's name and address, as they travel across the border. The Abortion Dream Team provides instructions via email and social media regarding how to take them, and volunteers are available to advise and answer questions throughout the process. The person taking the pills can also call the Abortion without Borders helpline to receive support from the Kobiety W Sieci team.

The Abortion Dream Team stays in touch after the pharmacological abortion is over too. "Usually, people want to go to the doctor to make sure everything is OK," explains Adrianna. "But the vagina is such a great organ that it will clear itself without even checking." She says people often write to the team afterward to thank it and express how happy they are. "The stigma of abortion is such a big thing in Poland, they usually cannot tell even their partners or friends. So I think the most important role we have is that we are giving the support. We are with you, you are not alone, and this is your decision. This is a good decision."

Activists in the Abortion without Borders network agree that the first thing that changed in the wake of Poland's near-total abortion ban was that an atmosphere of fear gripped doctors, nurses, and patients. Asia of Women Help Women observes that the most heartbreaking effect is that many people taking abortion pills are concerned they might not get adequate medical support in the event of complications, and that doctors might treat them as if they've committed a crime. Since the ban took effect in January 2021, at least three women have died of sepsis in Polish hospitals as a result of doctors refusing to perform a lifesaving abortion or caesarean section. "Someone who is taking abortion pills is not breaking the law," Asia says, "but doctors don't know it."

Coming from Poland's anarchist punk scene and queer feminist movement, Asia moved to Amsterdam to work with Women Help Women because of the limitations on what kind of support she could provide to those seeking abortions in Poland due to the legal restrictions. Women Help Women is a formal organization located in different areas around the world, but "we are not a huge organization," Asia explains. "We focus on the countries where there is not access to safe abortion services." Women Help Women also operates along a horizontal organizational culture, which Asia points out requires "constant conversation" about what it means to organize nonhierarchically. And "we try to change the narrative and promote a supportive, nonjudgmental, nor-malizing-of-abortion approach," she says.

All the collectives in the network share the goal of not only decriminalizing but also demedicalizing abortion. "Abortion pills are something that you can do on your own. You can decide when you want to have this abortion, how to do it," Adrianna underscores, noting that sadly, "like every area of life," people's decision-making power is frequently "taken by politicians or men in power."

"For me, this is actually the feminist revolution," says Asia. She explains that the idea of the procedure as something ethically controversial and prohibitively complicated is a construct that has nothing to do with reality. "It's not really about safety because the safety of it is proven. It's about control and keeping this atmosphere of dependency of people."

In Germany, one of the countries where Abortion without Borders helps people from Poland to access abortion services, the procedure is controlled by the state. While it is illegal to terminate a pregnancy in Germany, the law makes exceptions for medically necessary abortions and cases where the pregnancy is the result of rape. It also does not prosecute abortions in the first trimester, as long as people first submit to mandatory counseling with a state-licensed social worker (which laws require to be biased toward dissuading the person from having an abortion), followed by a compulsory three-day waiting period. Abortions in Germany can be surgical or pharmacological, but must always be performed in a clinic; one cannot simply order the pills and take them at home.

Ciocia Basia, the collective that supports people from Poland who choose to obtain abortions in Berlin, has always been small, informal, and self-organized, according to one member. It was initiated in 2015 by two people, one German and one Polish, who wanted to help bring people who were seeking abortions from Poland to the neighboring countries. The organizers started to make connections and formed their first partnership with a clinic that had affordable fees. After they began to receive phone calls from people in Poland seeking assistance, they decided to name the collective Ciocia Basia, which means "Auntie Basia" in Polish. Basia is a common name in Poland, so people can save the group's number on their phones without raising suspicion.

People in Poland seeking an abortion sometimes find Ciocia Basia through an article or interview in the course of searching for resources, or else through prochoice groups in Poland that distribute propaganda in the streets and media. One collective member reports that they try to be visible, going to demonstrations in Poland to pass out stickers and flyers. Every week, two members take regular shifts answering the phone number and email account via which people contact them. Once a person reaches out, members help them to decide whether coming to Germany for the procedure is an option. Ordering pills for a pharmaceutical abortion costs less money, so if this seems like a better route for the person, members refer them to the website for Women Help Women and stay involved in case they have questions.

Because Ciocia Basia strongly values self-determination, it is important that the pregnant person decide whether the abortion will be pharmacological or surgical, regardless of the practicalities for them or the group members. "We try not to put people with less or no money in the position where something is being decided for them only because their financial situation forces them to use our help," one member says.

The collective works with a network of people living in Berlin who host those coming to the city for an abortion. Collective members meet people at the train station and transport them to the place they will be staying, and from there to the clinic. According to one member, the activists don't host people themselves because it is too draining to be doing the logistical work as well. When someone needs a place to stay, members of the collective email a pool of volunteers to see who can host, explaining how many people will be coming and how many nights they need to stay, and hosts write back to answer whether they have room available. In some cases, Ciocia Basia pays for a hostel or simply directs people to hostels. The group also partners with volunteer translators to support those who don't speak German.

"We work as a grassroots collective with consensus decision-making process, task rotation, and some conflict resolution procedures," a member explains. "We have no formal hierarchy, and constantly try to notice and address the informal ones." The funding the group receives from local individual supporters covers all the costs of procedures, including transportation, allowing them to be financially independent. "In Berlin, people love organizing parties to raise funds and often approach us saying they want to do that for us, so we don't have to organize it by ourselves," they say. "This work requires having money, having access to money. You need many people so you don't get burned out. This is emotional work." Ciocia Basia practices collective care internally as well as externally. This manifests in bimonthly online meetings where "we try to check the workload, share the difficult moments. We also use chat in between the meetings. Taking a break is a common practice."

While a person still cannot be prosecuted for having an abortion in Poland, anyone who supports someone in obtaining one can, and the authorities appear to be sending a message to those who would do so. In November 2021, Abortion Dream Team cofounder Justyna Wydrzyńska became the first activist in Europe to face criminal charges for aiding an abortion. Justyna, who has been supporting people seeking abortions for fifteen years, sent a packet of abortion pills she had kept for her personal use to a woman who said her abusive partner was preventing her from leaving Poland to get the procedure. After the woman's partner found the package of pills and reported her and Justyna to the police, Justyna was arrested and faced up to three years in prison. The next year and a half saw the Abortion Dream Team, wider abortion rights movement, and human rights organizations such as Amnesty International rally behind her, afraid of the dangerous precedent a conviction in her case would set. On March 14, 2023, the Warsaw court convicted Justyna and sentenced her to thirty hours of community service a month for eight months, sparking outrage worldwide. Justyna's lawyers plan to appeal the verdict, while she and the Abortion Dream Team remain determined to continue their work to destigmatize abortion.

Despite these new developments and their ominous effects, proabortion activists in Poland remain encouraged by many people's response to the ban. "For me, what was really beautiful and mind-blowing was the solidarity organizing that happened after the court ruling," remarks Asia, "and people who started to declare that they did have abortions, they are willing to support others, they know how to do it. I feel like we need more and more of this, because it has such a power of destigmatizing the procedure itself and changing that narrative around it."

Adrianna maintains that creating networks is critical to this struggle. "I think in groups, we have power. You are not fighting alone. Even for me as an activist, I feel safer and that I have more possibilities when I'm in this network."

As these collectives continue to spread feminist anarchist ideals in the most powerful way possible—by demonstrating their effectiveness through action—members hope more and more people will take up the revolutionary work of meeting each other's needs directly. "I'm really impressed and grateful for the grassroots organizing that is happening around this topic, and I would love this to be spreading," says Asia. "Everyone can do it. It's so easy. All the information is there on the internet. Everyone can support someone with an unwanted pregnancy and how to terminate it. I really hope that people are going to take this opportunity to build more support networks for each other."

Regardless of what happens on the legislative front, the groups that comprise Abortion without Borders remain determined to continue their direct action. "The next step has to come soon; it is about the law change," notes a Ciocia Basia member. "The resources that the movement has or needs, however, will be still utilized—supporting people in late pregnancies, financial help, providing the information, educating, etc. We will not disappear from one day to another. And some of us will still have to face the repression. In this patriarchal, racist, and capitalistic society, you have to rest and recharge regularly, but you can't quit the resistance structures."

❖ ❖ ❖

Megan McGee is a writer and activist based in New York City who works with several mutual aid and community gardening initiatives. To read more of her work, please visit meganmcgee.com.

# TRANSITION AND AUTONOMY

## /

SCOTT/SHULI BRANSON

The lie is that centralized, state solutions are easy, efficient, and better in terms of supplying people with what they need. In truth, bureaucracy just keeps the messiness out of the spotlight—until you try to get something done. Then, alongside the direct violence of the state, one experiences death by a million paper cuts while trying to get insurance coverage, food stamps, unemployment, or name changes, or death by the abandonment of already unreliable resources. This is increasingly clear right now, as the state ups its attacks on bodily autonomy, using policies and courts to eviscerate trans-affirming care and abortion access.

As anarchists, in contrast, the way we do things—bottom up, not top down—is about *living*: how we choose to relate to each other, how we choose love and relationships over individualized endeavor and competition, how we choose to care even when that means working in the cracks and gray areas. Such "care work" is often done by feminized people, and as feminist organizers have long pointed out, frequently neglected, made invisible, or not seen as the real work of movements. Yet it is—and always has been—a crucial form of direct action, just as militant and risky as confronting police, fascists, and other coercive infrastructure in the streets.

In the current context, such direct action looks like informal networks of trans communities that get people hormones and take them to clinics, or regional abortion funds and doula collectives that get people abortions either at home or in a clinic. It's not merely *direct action* because these groups typically operate within the gray areas of the law, and not simply because the work is in confrontation with the current arms of the state trying to end bodily autonomy for trans people and pregnant people—though these are both good reasons to name it as such. Even more, this care work is direct action because it's operating outside the structures of the state in a prefigurative manner, outside the feelings of scarcity that the state imposes and anarchists themselves frequently reproduce.

Partially in response to the attack on access to trans-affirming care, then, and the general difficulty and expense of getting hormones through institutional medical channels, various groups across the so-called United States are making their own estrogen, whether topical, injectable, or oral. This isn't necessarily new. There's a history within trans communities of sharing hormones given that people's ability to procure them can be inconsistent based on insurance and finances. Currently, Boobs Not Bombs is one name given to decentralized networks of mutual aid groups making and distributing estrogen. And the Northeastern Fairy Wings chapter and other regional groups have recently written zines containing recipes for making your own estrogen at home, including options for sourcing the materials.

Estrogen is not a controlled substance, and so this DIY hormone process is ostensibly legal.[1] But with the generally hostile atmosphere toward trans people as well as the propensity of both the state and medical-industrial complex to get involved in regulating access and thus making it harder for people to care for themselves, the groups have deemed it best to call as little attention to themselves as possible—even as they attempt to form open points of access for any

---

1. Testosterone, on the other hand, is a controlled substance and therefore making it is illegal. It's possible that people are doing this, though, or finding black market testosterone.

trans person to have hormones. Groups are able to distribute six- to ten-month individual supplies at house shows, radical bookfairs and bookstores, community spaces, and more, along with pertinent information for making and taking hormones.

Using decentralized groups to make and distribute hormones helps respond to the general unevenness of access and attack state by state, since people in states with easier access and more room to maneuver can connect with groups in more oppressive states, thereby bypassing the restrictions. This model is replicable wherever people are, and so it's possible to keep multiplying the locations where hormones can be handed out, even in surprising places. That said, one organizer with Fairy Wings worries that "the distribution of DIY hormones could get stuck in subcultural spaces, like trans/anarchist/punk communities, which can leave out younger people in more highly surveilled family situations or states where access to care has been criminalized."

Still, even the possibility of DIY hormones can completely alter our understanding of transition. If hormones can be freely acquired outside the medical-industrial complex, then anyone can transition based on their own desires. This promise can help lessen the stigma around transition, which relies on pseudoscientific misinformation to back it up. Common discourse treats transition like an irreversible and potentially dangerous decision, even though in practice, people often go on and off hormones for various reasons. With groups like Boobs Not Bombs, someone could get a vial, tube, or bottle of estrogen, try it out, and figure out if it's what they want. Boobs Not Bombs follows the informed consent model, which is how precious few clinics that provide trans health care also work. Rather than needing a diagnosis, the person getting hormones is given information about potential risks and allowed to make their own decision. The Fairy Wings chapter includes links to further information about the best practices of taking estrogen in its zine, with extensive documentation for different questions. One of the members mentioned that trans patients and trans researchers usually know more than many medical gatekeepers about the science behind hormone therapy, and frequently have to educate their doctors about not only surgery and hormones but all aspects of their lives and bodies as well. Many doctors fall prey to the same misinformation and bad science that besets the general public. This misinformation within the medical-industrial complex is tied to profit too, and so doesn't produce good studies on trans care, whether because of a lack of interest/profitability or simply transphobia.

Like with abortion, transition has been individualized and privatized. The medicalized version of transition, which has become dominant, was developed to make it harder for people to do so in order to protect the liability of doctors against patients' potential regrets. It involves a person first finding a doctor who is willing to provide gender-affirming care such as hormones and surgeries. And even if one finds such a doctor, there are more obstacles to overcome in terms of proving to the caregiver that one is *really* trans (something there is no test for). This "proof" could be through diagnosis by a mental health professional, and used to involve the "real-life test" of living as your desired gender for a certain amount of time before being able to access hormones or surgery. Historically, people weren't only judged based on their fitting the diagnosis of transsexual as a medical and mental condition; they were often judged based on their willingness to participate in the reproduction of cisheterosexual norms in terms of how they dressed, whom they dated, and so on.

Just to say it again, because it bears repeating with different emphasis: with DIY hormones, anyone can transition whenever they want. This means you can experiment. It means you can stop. It means transition can become multiple, plural, and deindividualized. Not only can you access hormones in community with other trans people—something we have always done—but you can find more people and networks to run your questions by, and there's now more room to experiment. The groups are mainly oriented toward helping people find ways to replicate the production process on their own. Groups are also organizing communal shot-taking events, partially in response to the fear that some people have of injections and the need for support in administering them. Shots of testosterone and estrogen can be taken as part of ritual and celebration. And of course, this goes for other methods of receiving exogenous hormones too. When trans existence is under such extensive threat, these collective moments of transition are in themselves a direct action against the world that wants to erase us.

Though Fairy Wings specifically focuses on increasing access to free DIY estrogen, one member of the group with experience organizing community care thinks the model has wider implications: "We can collectively and intentionally think about what ways we actually need to rely on the medical system and what ways we don't, and solving as many problems as we can outside that. What contributes to people's health is mostly not doctors" but instead filling needs for housing, food, and freedom of movement, not to mention the relative health of air and water. Just as anarchist biohacking groups like the Four Thieves Vinegar Collective are spreading free mifepristone (a drug taken orally to induce abortion) and instructions on how to make it, there are collectives making insulin. A Fairy Wings member asks, "What if we had the ten most commonly used drugs readily available in a community pharmacy? This could reduce our reliance on state institutions, and remove points of contact with these institutions for people criminalized through race, gender, sexuality, citizenship, participation in sex work, and so on." Additionally, readily accessible medicines help us find communal care outside the privatized, isolated arrangements of normative families and couples.

Of course, we aren't currently in the position to do away with the medical system itself. Many people rely on complex medications embedded in present-day supply chains; others depend on medical equipment that is hard to manufacture. But it's simply a colonialist, ableist, scarcity, and antifeminist mentality that limits our revolutionary horizons from imagining ways to provide care to all who need it. Too much of the time, when we collectively envision liberated futures, disabled, trans, and chronically ill people are left behind, or erased altogether from the picture. In providing abortions, transition, and other medicines, collective care projects show us that we can take matters into our own hands. We can also imagine recruiting more scientists and doctors to help share knowledge and resources, and divert top-down institutional power toward increasing and disseminating access. Ultimately, as one comrade suggests, "we can dare to take over the hospitals and form people's clinics." And we'll need people who can help run them.

When it comes to abortion care, community clinics are something that abolitionist and abortion doula Ash Williams is thinking about. In the wake of the *Dobbs* decision that overturned *Roe v. Wade*, he has not wavered in his commitment to help anyone who wants an abortion to get one regardless of where it has to be done due to criminalization or how much it costs. While he acknowledges that "we need to fight to keep the existing clinics open," Ash asks, "What will it look like outside the clinic? ... I keep returning to the idea that the clinic isn't the best place for people to have an abortion." As Ash underscores, just as for trans care, the clinics are limited in what they perceive as medically relevant and therefore narrowly define best practices. Add to that the way that antiabortion and transphobic policies attack providers at the point of their liability, and so as to avoid punishment, many clinics overcompensate by limiting care. But even worse, the state in many cases has recruited providers, doctors, and nurses to inform on people who have abortions and/or access transition care. In fact, Ash contends that this threat might be one of the biggest dangers for people living in criminalizing states, over and beyond the actual police.

According to Ash, we can imagine and practice "models for access to care not governed by what the state says is legal or possible or medically relevant." We can create community abortion and transition clinics (if we want to continue using that word) that honor the autonomy and self-determination of the people seeking care, believing that people might be in the best position to decide for themselves what care they want. On the negative side, we're in a situation where, as Ash notes, "the state is failing to provide care," and even more so, we're seeing the "criminalization of the care that is being offered"—from criminalizing the act of doing an abortion and the support for those abortions, to criminalizing mutual aid efforts or the act of simply giving people free food or money in public, to criminalizing people trying to defend the earth, such as in the Stop Cop City movement in the Atlanta forest. So Ash warns that we need "to be mindful and skilled with the support that we give" so that we aren't merely giving care but instead offering "care and safety."

As Black feminist reproductive justice organizers tell us, *Roe* was never enough, and within a few years the Hyde Amendment limited federal resources for abortion, effectively making it inaccessible to all but the wealthy, thus disproportionately affecting Black women and other women of color. *Roe* was decided on the grounds of privacy, not bodily autonomy or collective care. This individualization of the issue helped spell its downfall. Similarly, the access to professional medical care for trans people was dictated by the doctors who deigned to treat trans people as an individualized matter, with significant trials and obstacles put up to make sure that only a few people could access hormones or surgery (and limit liability for any hypothetical regrets people would have after transition).

Both in the struggle for reproductive autonomy and trans care, there is an unwritten and continuous legacy of organizing that occurs out of the spotlight. The most well-known historical examples might be the Jane Collective, an underground network of women in Chicago from 1969 to

1973 that performed over ten thousand abortions during that time, and the Street Transvestite Action Revolutionaries, a short-lived group formed by Sylvia Rivera and Marsha P. Johnson that worked toward the survival of young trans street kids of color and sex workers, particularly by forming the STAR House, a communal living space. These two (trans) feminist action groups emerged during the height of the liberation movements of the long 1960s, and along with the decline and repression of those movements, the visibility of radical experiments faded in the neoliberal blur of draining state resources, increased policing and incarceration, and a worsening daily grind of mere survival. These are the times we live in now, surrounded by constant reminders that climate catastrophe is here, not in some near future. Many of us today look at these earlier groups with admiration and perhaps even envy that they were able to pull off such powerful actions.

When the major talking points around issues like abortion or hormones and surgery now focus on individual access, we can easily overlook the communal impact of the assaults on bodily autonomy: the isolation, fear, and mistrust that arises, and loss of comrades from burnout, despair, or worse. One major difference between us organizers today and the collectives of the 1960s and 1970s is the further atomization of communities in general, along with a heightened sense of scarcity for survival. But the relative lack of attention on communal forms of underground organizing has also allowed groups to work, and with good success, in the cracks. Abortion funds and doula collectives raise money, give people rides to clinics—even across state lines—distribute medical abortions, and provide the emotional support that pregnant people need when considering terminating a pregnancy. Trans groups raise money for surgeries and basic daily needs, make and distribute or share hormones, get people to their appointments, support trans people who are incarcerated, and create new rituals together.

Working in the cracks often draws criticism for supposedly further enabling the neoliberal withdrawal of resources. And indeed, sometimes the state doesn't criminalize mutual aid but rather commends it for helping people in areas where the state has clearly failed. Yet the mutual aid direct action groups providing abortions and hormones are doing something beyond filling the gaps and enabling the system to continue on its pathway toward megadestruction. They crack open the professionalization and medicalization of care, including abortion and transition, and aid us in glimpsing a reorganization of what care might look like—offering a transfeminist and anarchistic alternative.

Boobs Not Bombs, Fairy Wings, abortion doula collectives, and other "gray area" projects, alongside all else they do, contribute to expanding our sense of care beyond these immediate criminalized efforts, making sure that we include disabled people, chronically ill people, youths and children, parents, incarcerated people, unhoused people, sex workers, and more—people who currently have to organize their own alternatives to the dominant forms of care. In this wisdom are the seeds for growing better networks. We can use the patchwork of the state as we need right now, while organizing for a takeover through decentralized groups that prioritize the people receiving care in determining their own needs through mutualistic direct action.

* * *

Scott/Shuli Branson is a queer/transfemme Jewish anarchist writer, translator, community organizer, and teacher. They translated Jacques Lesage de la Haye's *The Abolition of Prison* and Guy Hocquenghem's second book of essays, *Gay Liberation after May '68*, for which they also wrote a critical introduction on his queer anarchism. She coedited *Surviving the Future: Abolitionist Queer Strategies* with Raven Hudson and Bry Reed for PM Press. Shuli is the author of *Practical Anarchism: A Guide for Daily Life* and is currently working on a book on trans youth liberation. They often contribute to the Final Straw Radio, a weekly anarchist radio show and podcast. Her new project is a talk show called "The Breakup Theory," where anarchists and queers discuss the ways their politics show up in their relationships. Scott is grateful for the comrades who shared their experiences, wisdom, and time to support the report back in this essay.

# MOVEMENT MIDWIFERY

# /

## VICKY OSTERWEIL

The most beautiful thing I ever saw does not, to my knowledge, have any photographic record. It was early in the morning, some weekday in mid-July 2018. It was an hour before my shift doing data entry in a big office building in Center City, Philadelphia, giving me time to check in with the OccupyICE encampment outside City Hall. When I arrived that morning, however, I didn't find the mess of police barricades, improvised kitchen equipment, propaganda and handwritten signs, plastic totes, and trash bags as well as bedding arranged underneath the massive, dumpstered billboards we used as canopy.

Instead, I saw a forest.

The night before, the city had done some landscaping around City Hall, and the activists who were occupying full time had gathered branches and other refuse, then lovingly arranged them on, inside, and across the city's traffic bollards and barricades, in and through the tents, poles, and tables. Early morning sunlight diffused through the fog rising from the concrete after a light summer rain. Though it was already after 7:00 a.m., the camp was slumbering peacefully as I entered this suddenly ethereal, unfamiliar space.

In the shadow of the enormous monument to state power that is Philadelphia City Hall, under a jerry-rigged awning made from the city's garbage and offcuts, the "disposable" and dispossessed had built a grove, a space of clean air, beauty, safety, and love; they had transformed thirty feet of pavement into a garden for deep sleep. I started to cry. I knew that we could win.

But few people were allowed this vision. Philly mayor Jim Kenney had declared himself against Immigration and

Customs Enforcement (ICE) and Donald Trump, and wasn't ready to give up the public pretense to #resistance, so he had agreed that if we didn't block sidewalk traffic, the police wouldn't interfere with our encampment. Until the eviction, he broke this promise exactly once: that morning. The cops forced the encampment to take down the forest. The sight of liberation terrifies the police.

The upsurge of movement, solidarity, and organizing across the 2010s accelerated in anxiety and urgency under Trump. The George Floyd Rebellion looms large over the entire decade, but even the airport shutdowns, antifascist militancy, Indigenous resistance, mutual aid, org building, and prison struggles of those years overshadow the OccupyICE movement.

The movement—in which activists encircled and built street occupations around urban ICE headquarters in an attempt to shut down that distinctly American gestapo—appeared in over a dozen cities, yet even its longest-running incarnations were over within a few months of their appearance. The tactic of tent-based occupations seemed to emerge out of the past, as both its promises and limits had been thoroughly met in the "Movement of the Squares" cycle of 2011–14, and policing and state agencies had a good idea of how to counter this movement style.

But the movement is more than just a footnote in a decade of struggle, at least here in Philadelphia. OccupyICE not only won a major concession from the city—the end of the information-sharing agreement between city bureaucracies and ICE known as PARS; it also forged a community of unhoused organizers and housing advocates that would go on to seed a number of future movements in the city. And trans women—both housed and unhoused—played the crucial role in keeping OccupyICE going.

After weeks of planning, a coalition of radical groups in Philadelphia held a rally outside City Hall on July 2, 2018. Hundreds showed up, marching to ICE offices at Eighth and Cherry Streets, where an occupation was spontaneously set up. At first protesters barricaded the streets around the building, but the organizers, who seemed surprised by the success of the demonstration, negotiated with the police to take down the blockade and remain on the sidewalk. This moment, in which activists in high-visibility vests were seen dismantling the barricades at the cops' demand—and an altercation between the "official" organizers and anarchists frustrated by their action—was a sign of things to come. Still, the space was held, and an occupation with tents and umbrellas was established, blocking ICE.

The days that followed were marked by intense heat, police violence, eviction attempts, and increasingly hostile sectarian conflict, both between anarchists and socialists (anarchists were physically ejected from the camp by socialists because they refused to take off their masks and then published a pamphlet calling the socialist organizers wannabe cops) as well as within the encampment, where democratic processes were never initiated and power devolved upward to the "experienced" organizers.

When, on July 5, police came in swinging clubs, making arrests, and destroying what was left of the encampment infrastructure, the movement's energy seemed spent, and there was little fight left to rebuild.

That might have been the end of it, except that a group of autonomous activists had constructed the beginnings of a new encampment ten blocks away, on the sidewalk outside City Hall. This new encampment featured no high-vis vests and few of the organizers of the original demo. Many of the initial organizers were burned out, and while they continued to have meetings (and fundraise for themselves!) around OccupyICE, they were basically absent from this second camp.

Instead, a steady trickle of folks, housed and unhoused, started to gather daily and build out this new encampment. The organizers of this new encampment were majority Black and unhoused, and a surprisingly high percentage of the activists, housed and unhoused, white and Black, were trans femmes and nonbinary people.

The City Hall encampment never reached the numbers or resources of the previous one, and I wasted much of my own time trying to get the originating orgs to see that the movement continued, going to endless meetings in their spaces, offering good faith encouragements, and attempting to develop relationships—all to no avail. These orgs only came back to the camp in force once, on the day that Mayor Kenney announced the end of PARS—for a photo op. I would find out months later that the entire time, the initial organizers were talking shit in Facebook groups and Signal threads, and cravenly continuing to accept donations raised on the backs of the activism of Black unhoused trans folks. So much for today's would-be Lenins.

On the ground, though, over the span of a couple of weeks, the encampment went through a slow but steady transformation from the kind of chaotic, service-oriented structure that would be familiar to people who've worked in nonprofit-type movement efforts, into an intensely politicized space of immigrant solidarity and resistance. Many young and idealistic organizers, well-intentioned yet unconsciously bringing these nonprofit models of activism, couldn't deal with the concentrated "drama" of drug use, explosive conflicts, mental health crises, criminal proximities, and difficult personalities, and dropped out. But sticking through it all, a handful of organizers, mostly trans femmes and nonbinary folks, did the unseen and uncelebrated work of weaving a community out of a group of angry and dispossessed people.

A trans woman bottom-lined the kitchen, streamlining both donation acceptance and meal prep with the help of an unhoused person in their twenties who would go on to transition herself after her experience in the movement, which she cited as inspiring her to do so. Another trans woman, only recently housed and personally familiar with many of the folks living at the camp, acted as a de facto conflict moderator and de-escalator. A third girl, with the help of other activists, filled a table with propaganda, and encouraged a focus on political language and messaging to passersby in this central downtown location—a task joyfully taken up by a few unhoused folks, one elder woman in particular, who spent hours on a megaphone and quickly became a lead organizer in the group. A nonbinary organizer began holding and facilitating meetings in the camp, while two other nonbinary folks took regular dumpster diving trips for materials to expand the physical infrastructure.

Without this queer community-building, this movement midwifery, through which a collection of troubled, societally disadvantaged, and oppressed folks turned into a fighting force, the encampment at City Hall would not have survived. Instead, within two weeks, it had become a space from which direct actions—including street-taking marches, antifascist interventions, and support marches for other activist groups working in the city—emerged "spontaneously." And the movement grew strong enough to force the mayor's hand, compelling him to acquiesce to the demand that the city end its data sharing with ICE. In 2020, organizers who met through OccupyICE would found the unhoused encampments that would capture significant numbers of houses and resources from the Philadelphia Housing Association, and help change the face of housing politics in the city—encampments that were once again disproportionately supported and organized by trans folks.

This exhausting and thankless reproductive labor is one of the core concerns of feminist theory and action. But in spaces of the multiply marginalized and dispossessed, trans and gender-nonconforming folks' capacity to "stay with the trouble," as feminist scholar Donna Haraway puts it, often facilitates the completion of this labor.[1] This capacity is frequently hard-won through the experience of transness, both internally and socially.

To hold onto a truth that bosses, families, and friends want to question or reject, that doctors and the state want to medicalize and control, a truth that goes against your own intense internalized distrust, ignorance, misinformation, and transphobia, and to still come out and be your fabulous self

---

1. Donna J. Haraway, *Staying with the Trouble: Making Kin in the Chthulucene* (Durham, NC: Duke University Press, 2016).

requires an ability to fight through a great thicket of contradictory and confusing needs and desires. To hold your pre- and posttransition experiences as your own personal experiences, to be able to code switch, pass, or stealth as survival and personal circumstances require, to have a clear vision of gendered experiences and expectations that are entirely invisible to the vast majority of cis people, who likely as not treat you like you're paranoid or crazy for recognizing them, in fact to be blamed both within queer and activist communities as well as the greater world for the existence of these contradictions—this is the psychic burden of transphobia and gender on us.

And while this horrific psychic violence is a travesty that our struggle aims to abolish, it also gives many of us a wisdom, persistence, strength, and power of insight that although it came at much too great a cost, can be used to help others go through the confusing and difficult processes of personal change, growth, and transformation. The trans person knows, better than anyone, that we can only act from where we stand, that what we say, do, and know to be true can shape the world around us, but only if we get our hands dirty in the messy facts of everyday life.

Trans people are thus particularly attuned to holding space for people's pain, exhaustion, contradictory tendencies, and even reactionary views; not giving up on struggles or movements because they fail to emerge fully formed and perfect; hanging onto a truth in the face of repression, disagreement, and incongruities; and fighting for that truth while bringing others alongside them in the fight. Trans anarchic feminism takes the offcuts, prunings, and refuse of this world, and makes a beautiful forest for our flourishing, pleasure, rest, and joy.

At the moment of this writing, in 2023, trans people are organizing hormone exchanges, DIY medical support, abortion access, and logistical networks to get trans folks out of US states and cities dominated by transphobic policies. But these practices have long existed in our communities, here and elsewhere; they've simply become more urgent, more visible, and more organized. And while these movements and groups may be easier to name as "trans feminism," trans women have been at the center of all the movements of the last decade, quietly practicing the world-building that will abolish this terrible nightmare we find ourselves in. That world will be built bric-a-brac from the products of this one, through a movement that recognizes the possibilities inherent in all of us, and promises, slowly, carefully, but fearlessly, to bring out such beauty that the police, bootlickers, patriarchs, and fascists will run, terrified, from our irresistibly radiant freedom.

❖   ❖   ❖

This essay is dedicated to Jennifer Bennetch (1985–2022), who inspired and changed everyone she struggled beside. May her memory be a revolution.

Vicky Osterweil is a writer, worker, and agitator based out of Philadelphia. She is the author of two books: *In Defense of Looting* (Bold Type, 2020) and *The Extended Universe* (Haymarket, 2024).

# HOW WE PERSISTED AS
# A NEW ANARCHA GROUP
# IN LJUBLJANA

/

ČRNE MAČKE

*How to write a collective reflection in a place without electricity during a time when we'd run out of wood for our heater and our car-battery-powered lights were constantly, slowly dying out.*

## HOW IT STARTED

In 2020, some parts of the antiauthoritarian movement in slovenia (re-, re-, re)recognized the need to create space to address feminist issues more thoroughly.[1] At the time, the clerofascist government had taken power after the previous prime minister resigned just as the COVID epidemic was declared in our territory. Different groups and individuals (anarchists, communists, various antigentrification fronts, and the two ljubljana squats in existence then) came together at an assembly to form an anticapitalist bloc and call for a broader mobilization to join in protests every Friday. Through these mobilizations, we, the anticapitalists, saw the opportunity to focus on issues that extended further but also correlated with the rise of fascism around us. We addressed deadly neoliberal politics, the ineffectiveness of the state's health care system, the ever-so-aggravated and volatile impending ecological armageddon, and the rise of wars and conflicts around the globe.

At this same assembly, people decided that the anticapitalist bloc should write and release a statement about the antiabortion situation in poland, and a working group was created to carry out the task. We don't remember if it was a coincidence (probably it wasn't), but the group that formed was all female. After the statement was written, our working

---

1. As part of our anarcha-feminist practice, we lowercase words that currently have hierarchical power in the world, such as the names of cities, nation-states, and geopolitical regions.

group felt the urge to meet more often among ourselves. So we circled up to reflect on feminist topics together as well as offer each other emotional support as women involved in anarchist struggles. We sat together drinking tea and talking about everything from our broader organizing efforts along with our own need for separate actions and involvement, but also highly personal issues relating to relationship trauma, sexual harassment, reproductive health with an emphasis on our distrust of the gynecology field, and our witchy self-help tricks and tips.

Soon we recognized the need to take our discussion circle to the level of organized activism. We quickly engaged in our first action, from which our first "solo" statement arose, and decided to sign it as "črne mačke" (black cats). Almost immediately, though, some of our comrades confronted us, asking what it meant that we'd signed this statement as a group. Some people offered arguments against us being able to call ourselves a name that appeared to be a collective because we were as they called us "a newly formed initiative." Most of the mansplaining about what the differences of a group, collective, and initiative are came from our male comrades. We felt like it was an attempt to discourage us from forming something we believed was going to last. We retaliated: we decided to keep the name and not be forced to explain the status of our newly formed coalition of anarcha-feminists looking for our own space to be able to organize.

We kept exploring issues that we felt were not being addressed through the broader mobilization, which we are all still very much a part of to this day. We dedicated banner drops, statements, protests, and demonstrations to the issues of rape, sexual harassment, femicides, the church, and antiabortion movements, but also to struggles against the elites, gentrification, wars, apartheid, and border regimes. We continued to concentrate on anticapitalist and antistatist efforts, yet through the lens of fighting patriarchy, which we see as the basis of our oppression.

## SPACE

In the beginning, črne mačke gathered on the second floor of the Autonomous Factory Rog in a small space that had been occupied and renovated by one of our members, who made it into a cozy hideout for witches and herbalists. On the rooftop of this squat, she'd set up a small garden and always provided self-picked teas for our meetings.

At 7:00 a.m. on January 19, 2021, in the midst of a cold winter and during the peak of the second wave of the COVID pandemic, the municipality of ljubljana along with support of the police decided to violently evict the Autonomous Factory Rog. The loss of this huge factory space meant that a lot of groups now found themselves displaced in the city. New self-organized spaces seemed impossible to establish given that the police and security guards were controlling every step of those who did not obey the government's COVID restrictions, which were mostly just a pretext for imposing authoritarian policies rather than protecting the populace. This hostile environment prevented us from gathering and traveling. After the eviction, the city authority and private property owners even began to control and protect abandoned buildings from potential squatters.

All over the region, squats had already started disappearing in the years prior to the demolition of Rog, and specifically in ljubljana, which in recent years became a tourist hub. The city has been transformed by tourism. Profits became priority number one. Prices of living spaces went up, and the city center switched from focusing on the needs of its inhabitants to catering to tourists. Alternative venues that offered entertainment for visitors got municipal support, and of course many of those spaces eventually went mainstream in order to survive. The lack of autonomous space became a big problem, not just for us, but the wider community as well.

For a while, then, we didn't have a stable organizing place, until some comrades from an anarchist collective offered to let us share their space. Coexisting in what felt like the only radical spot left in gentrified ljubljana was not always easy, and led to multiple conflicts and tensions. We were extremely grateful for the existence of that place, and still are, but soon we realized that we needed to open a new squat. It took a while. At the time, we were still dealing with the aftermath of the Rog eviction and trying to cultivate good relations with our new hosts/roommates while fighting for our own space in what frequently felt like a manarchist place.

# MAČJAK

A year and a half after losing our beloved Autonomous Factory Rog, we changed the locks on an empty building, now known as mačjak. Mačjak offered us an opportunity to learn how to build a space from the ground up on our own terms and liberate ourselves from the previous arrangements. Opening a squat allowed us to become more autonomous, have space to think collectively, apply tactics we'd already developed, and establish new ones to solve problems we identified within the system and our movement.

Occupying mačjak changed a lot for us. It gave us independence from the collective that we shared the previous space with. It supplied us with new confidence to organize exactly how we wanted to, without the need for or feeling like we had to explain ourselves to anyone. It gave us a fresh perspective on power dynamics, putting us in the position of having a space and deciding whom to invite to organize in it. This not only influenced our relationships on the outside but also on the inside, within us. Since opening mačjak, we still struggle with the distribution of the care work that has to be put into the space and our collective. As a previously more or less street-oriented collective, we sometimes feel impatient and stuck when most of our energy is used for maintaining a place, sometimes leaving little capacity for outside actions.

One of the important questions related to mačjak was the notion of safe space—safe for whom, and from whom. Collectively we never felt comfortable with understanding safety on the basis of identity. Our struggle against patriarchy, which has always been at the core of our organizing, and later on "moving away" from the "oh so united anarchist movement against all forms of oppression" that sometimes couldn't recognize (and reflect on) its own sexist patterns, was read as a separatist move. So we decided to claim separatism as one of our strategies. We decided to define mačjak as an anarcha-queer space based on zero tolerance for sexism, machismo, racism, xenophobia, and any other forms of discriminatory tendencies. The basis of organizing in mačjak is therefore in political affinity, not some essentialist identity.

## HOW TO ORGANIZE

In the two years since we formed, our collective has gone through numerous changes in ideology and group dynamics, which sometimes we've tackled well and sometimes less effectively. As a feminist group, we are "experts" in self-care and excellent reproductive workers, yet we keep failing when trying to put these ideas into practice.

Looking at already established anarchist and feminist groups in our geographies, we felt that the first didn't recognize the importance of antisexist work, and the latter adopted neoliberal approaches in their fight against (gender) oppression. That's why we decided at first to forge our own organizing path based on our own values, wants, and capacities, and not focus too much on how to connect with other groups from the start.

Yet when there were fractures within our collective, and especially after we lost a number of members, we decided not to aim at expanding, even though we keep returning to this question at different points in our organizing. As a small group, it's easier to address conflicts and find common ground. Trust can be built and tended to more easily. We seek to find ideological consensus between ourselves while concentrating on what it means in terms of our social relations with each other to stick together as a working collective, including so we can always also reach out for support when the time comes or when we want to organize more broadly.

So far, we've managed to point out many structures and behaviors we don't want to reproduce among ourselves and our movements. We've noticed that even in radical circles, especially at assemblies, people are "forced" to develop patriarchal patterns to be accepted and respected. Having to be loud and articulate to be heard and taken seriously are some of those attitudes that we want to question. Being patient with people who can't form their opinions quickly, encouraging those who do not speak often, and leaving space are some of the strategies we want to further develop. We aim to recognize and dismantle informal hierarchies, not be competitive with each other, to actively listen, and to be able to take critique as a sign of growth. Many times, we've noticed that certain ideas are not questioned at all, since the person bringing them up has an already established position within the movement. If questioning occurred, it was some-times taken personally or even defensively, and instead of providing arguments for the idea, the person would defend their own ego, not wrestle generatively together with ways of how to move forward. We decided to take a stance against individualism because we feel that a person's political prestige has no place in collective organizing. So we're experimenting with new forms of collectivity, because the established ways of doing things and perspectives within our circles sometimes have to be questioned in order to reveal new ways of thinking and praxis suited to the times and challenges we face.

## FEMINISTS ON DUTY

When engaged in organizing beyond our collective in various struggles, we've often felt like the "feminists on duty." When there was an issue connected to abortion or rape, for instance, it was assigned to us; when addressing war, it was not assumed that we would even be interested. We recognize, however, that war and its repercussions have an inherently feminist dimension. Macho traits like pride in connection to patriotism, physical strength, and its association with weapons, competition, and binarism are all features that drive people to start wars or join armies in the first place. We see it as necessary to talk about "nonconventional" weapons used during wars, such as rape. On the practical side, there is a need to maintain spaces where people who desert and flee can find shelter; there is much care work to be done for people who've experienced war and the violence connected to it, not to mention dealing with rape victims.

While we see broader societal issues such as war through the lens of patriarchy, we also look at "typical" feminist themes through the lens of other hierarchical systems. For example, access to abortion in slovenia cannot be seen as just an individualist, liberal issue of "my body, my choice." The right to abortion is (for now) guaranteed, with some exceptions that can be tied to a range of capitalist and nationalist rationales. Even though abortion is considered basic health care in slovenia, people who do not have the right papers that the state imposes can't access it freely. Meaning that lots of people on the move or those who are seeking asylum are excluded, and even with the "correct" citizenship, abortion and health care aren't as self-evident to access as it might seem. Lately, too, finding a personal doctor is like looking for a needle in a haystack—especially for younger adults. To be able to abort, you must have a personal gynecologist or otherwise you need to pay for it (and not such a small amount for most of us).

## WE HAVE TO STAY OPEN

From our beginnings onward, we've questioned the women-only constellation and romanticized the idea of being viewed as a queer collective, even though we as collective members are generally read as heteronormative women by those who do not know us personally. One of the reasons why we opted for the queer label was also not to push away potential members who didn't identify as women. Yet this turned out to be not only an ideological struggle but a generational one too. We've been influenced in our thinking and organizing by different streams of oppressed peoples' movements—from our sisters organizing for women's rights in the balkan region, to our western comrades experimenting with living together in squats and housing projects, and from historical revolutionary movements to the more recent ones. Our older members have taken more inspiration from Indigenous women's struggles on other continents, while our younger ones relate more to the queer movements here in europe. We've all drawn inspiration from the Rojava women's autonomous organizing, and thus have embraced the need for women-only and all-oppressed-genders or FLINTA (female, lesbian, intersex, trans, and agender) groups, believing that they can coexist in parallel with mixed-group organizing, while also supporting men-only configurations within our movement.

We've tried and continue to strive for ways to establish a broader feminist platform that would involve as many people as possible in addressing social issues through a feminist lens. Should that be a general meeting, gathering, or communication channel? We're still not sure. For a while, we were involved in intergenerational feminist meetings, and after that we tried to have an open feminist gathering by inviting our friends, colleagues, and other people close to us who might be interested in feminist organizing. We also invited those who hadn't organized before. The outcomes of our efforts were always a bit different than planned, but still, a wider platform for organizing on feminist issues has formed, and there's now another active feminist collective here in ljubljana.

We are aware that oppressed groups of people frequently need to first establish space on their own to empower themselves and be able to organize without their oppressors, including as preparation to act as a stable group within a larger movement. But it is still an open question for us: how to develop and sustain our politics while creating a collaborative space for all oppressed persons. At this point in our growth process, we're involved with a FLINTA initiative that centers mainly on issues related to feminism, and we host a critical masculinity group. We host meetings and assemblies that are mixed in an attempt to connect our separate struggles and establish a mutual support system in our little city.

Through the process of writing this short reflection, a lot has changed for us.

We were confronted by our younger comrades about what they feel are generational hierarchies based on experience. We were challenged about various aspects of being gatekeepers of a space we tried to make and keep open for our sisters. We struggled with dynamics within our own collective and in connection with other collectives. We fought our declining mental health—some of us together, and others on their own.

We traveled and met people, and hosted groups and individuals here in our space that inspired us. We organized assemblies, protests, and direct actions on different topics. We failed to find the time and energy to keep new initiatives and projects going, and neglected care work. We started and quit jobs, finished our studies and started studying other topics, started new relationships and ended old ones. We made mistakes and tried to fix them. We left projects that frustrated us and moved away from struggles that overwhelmed us. We connected with groups that fell apart. We lost contacts, saw networks dying and could not find the energy to maintain them, and yet also formed new connections.

We felt excited. We got tired and burned out. We got arrested. We put ourselves and others in danger. We were sometimes depressed, and at other times manic. We were happy, and in other moments, disappointed. We hosted parties and concerts. We felt alive. We felt like our organizing was pointless. We hosted a big international event. We opened a new squat for our comrades from different territories and found space to connect again. We gave and felt love. We saw the point again. We reflected. We retaliated.

We persisted.

❊  ❊  ❊

črne mačke is a fairly new collective in ljubljana, slovenija. Its members represent a new generation, with little knowledge of the history of feminist or anarchist organizing in their city. They often felt alone until they started to create broader platforms for organizing on feminist and anarchist issues. You can get in touch with them over email: crnemacke@riseup.net.

# DO YOU FEEL THE SAME?

## /

VILJA SAARINEN

To all who share food, water, cigarettes, and tips and tricks with those in need.

To the ones who warn their fellow passengers when seeing ticket inspectors waiting on the metro platforms or stall the inspectors so as to gift the ones who haven't bought a ticket more time to get away.

To all who move closer to each other in the hope of becoming a territory.

To the parents who bring their kids to demonstrations. To everyone who waits outside jails and hospitals. To those who study first aid, law, and trauma support. To all who show up in the streets when it's below minus-15 degrees Celsius.

To anyone who has housed, hidden, and helped refugees, or arranged transport for them.

To everyone who has ever brought food or other treasures to collective spaces so that everyone could eat. Anyone who has peeled tens of kilograms of potatoes, fried hundreds of falafel, or organized places to meet, discuss, and learn. Saved plates of food for the ones who have not yet returned safely. Prepared meals separately for comrades with allergies. Invested in collective infrastructure. Been on a hunger strike.

To all of those caring for collective needs or doing the right thing even though it is risky.

To all that grows under the ice in the absence of sunshine.

To those struggling to unlearn patriarchy, moving back to give space, offering care, and moving forward in their work of understanding their emotions.

To Danuta, Tess, and all of you standing face-to-face with fascists, cops, or other violent men and not backing down.

To all of those who still carry the new world in their hearts.

To whoever has read this far.

I hope this letter finds you well.

I am writing to you in the desire that you will share a moment of cheerful nostalgia with me. When the times are difficult, to say the least, I sometimes try to get ahold of what put us on this path in the first place and why. It helps me feel closer to the things that make my heart beat a bit faster. It helps me feel closeness to you. Perhaps you remember the feeling that we shared when going to the first demonstration after a spring of quarantining and worrying about COVID-19, expecting a crowd of three hundred, but being greeted by three thousand. The feeling of something ice cold slowly melting. Like when I think back on the memory of Riikka stealing the hat of an infamous racist YouTuber and then tripping when running away, yet nevertheless making it to safety, it still evokes a whole range of emotions in me. A little fear, and a lot of joy and laughter. There is so much to be done. A lot has already happened.

I have some confessions to make. I am secretly impressed by the determination of the schoolgirl who sat alone in front of the Parliament to protest climate change until she wasn't alone anymore, and hundreds of thousands of kids and teenagers all around the world joined her. I love all the kids who got inspired, especially the five-year-olds in Tampere, carrying picket signs of animals facing extinction, depicting animals the same size as them. I love each and every one of you!

I adore the grandmas and grandpas who were among the first to climb the riot fence in Göteborg in 2017, after which almost ten thousand people followed their lead and blocked the route of the Nazi march. I still feel touched when I see the pictures from that day, just as I feel moved every time I watch the different "Un violador en tu camino" videos from many continents after the Chilean feminist collective Las Tesis created this song and dance, and it spread around the globe along with its final line, "The rapist is you!" With these street performance-protests, you really managed to show the world that when it comes to patriarchy, no one is innocent, and everyone should take the time to analyze their own behavior as well as the institutions around them and then act accordingly. And I get a warm feeling thinking of Nelli throwing the ripe tomato—with the proficiency of someone who has done nothing but throw tomatoes all of her life—that hit the Nazi leader on the head at the perfect second in front of a big crowd in Turku.

To this day, I can still recall the words of the Johannesburg Fees Must Fall activist who even when behind bars, said that the future looks so bright, he needs sunglasses. That attitude is something one needs in order to find the courage of the fifteen or so women who protested in front of a march of sixty thousand nationalists and fascists in Poland. I hope to one day gather enough faith and reckless abandon to follow their example, if the situation comes to that.

Love from Helsinki to Hong Kong to the persons who first tried to put out a tear gas grenade with a traffic cone, and all the others who continued tirelessly after that; you will go down in history. Love to the kids bloc in Malmö, the mom bloc in Portland, and all the tractor blocs ever.

Loukanikos, you wild riot dog, you took everything to a new level on the streets of Greece and put a big smile on our faces worldwide. May you rest in power! I wish a lot of smelly sausages, befitting your nickname, for you wherever you are! We will make sure that the memory of you outlasts the companies making the tear gas that weakened your lungs. Loldiers of Odin, you wild clowns, you managed to put an even bigger smile on our faces while sticking by migrants in Finland, and without cute animals at that. It's quite an achievement in today's online world, where cats reign supreme.

I salute the no-longer-captive beavers who built a tunnel to break out of the Ähtäri Zoo. I also salute the humans who follow the principle of "be water," most likely utterly unaware of these beavers.

On a sunny day in 2015 when people in Istanbul disobeyed the ban on the Pride parade and the police attacked them with water cannons, the sun and water created a rainbow over the protesters. That moment! That moment is when you know that not only your friends will have your back but also the universe itself. In that same spirit, I send warm thoughts the way of the neighbors who put up red signs on their doors in Hamburg during the G20 to show where protesters could find solidarity. The red signs were not in the shape of hearts per se but they were hearts nonetheless.

Just as I have tried to share some special memories with you, I hope you will take the time to think back on the situations when you felt collective dignity and strength. When your mind and gut screamed with excitement. Remember them, and embrace your desire for more. In our neighborhood, and on a planetary scale.

As friends have pointed out, we're like a mix of magnificent things that those working against us have difficulty understanding. They can't imagine fierceness and care inhabiting the same person, much less a social body that fights to dismantle hierarchies according to ethical principles of shared power. Love is not keeping your hands clean; love is courage.

When an event with people with strollers and walkers gets attacked, anyone who rushes to absorb the first blows and actively defend them, despite the consequences that might continue for one, two, four, seven, or even ten years, is defending love.

Anyone who dances Kurdish *halay* to keep up spirits and calm their friends while the police search their bus, home, or squat do so with an air of elegant resistance. *Zap, zap, zapê*!

But to be honest, the other reason I am writing to you is because it becomes more and more clear to me every day that we belong together, in one way or another. And I want you to remember that even though you sometimes, and perhaps often, feel lonely, you are loved!

I am certain of this. I know it deep down.

That is why I am writing to you, from the many places where I know it to be true. From the moments and movements where I have experienced and felt it to be true. Love as a constant practice.

From the floor of my house where I frequently lay down to gather strength and where I am now thinking of you. A floor that has supported so many others too.

From the friend, who happens to get their hands on two hundred vegan pizzas and calls to ask if you'd like some, and you feel that it's not only your political productivity that matters but that your body is being cared for too.

From the streets, every time you shout the chant *"Jin! Jiyan! Azadî!* / Women! Life! Freedom!" and you feel humble in the face of history and grateful for the path that is opening, on which you can journey with a bit more dignity.

From the eight-year-old who taught us a TikTok dance to the tune of the antifascist "Bella Ciao." Ylva, you are right, any event or revolution needs dancing, and we are honored to dance with you.

From the hangout after the biweekly meeting in spring 2020 where we first heard about what was going on in Seattle. When you made Capitol Hill an autonomous zone, it made us feel something we haven't felt in a long time, something we can't quite formulate yet. Not to mention the sacking of the Third Precinct in Minneapolis.

From the comradeship that can start to deepen through direct and honest communication. When we develop and dare to use tools and structures to solve, and even more important, prevent conflicts that cause crises in our communities, long-term relationships can begin to take shape.

From the care given by one to many, such as from Oscar, who regularly brought home, washed, and folded the towels of a shared social space for five years, without being asked to do it. We see the work you do and we love you.

From the meeting in the woods that becomes possible when the equipment from a juicery is repurposed into a field kitchen to cater for eighty people. First you learn to cook for two people. Then fifteen, a hundred, and even six thousand new friends.

From the territory that starts to form when Taneli from the other radical space in the neighborhood pops in and asks if he can clean our windows, and we catch the first glimpse of the love that will surround us when we inhabit the whole neighborhood instead of two little storefronts. Taneli, we wish we would have had more than decent coffee and enthusiastic visions to offer you in return.

From writing you this letter, and rereading our beautiful shared history of resistance and compassion. From noticing that I miss you and wondering what you're up to. In the words of our friends, organizing ourselves has never been anything else than loving each other.

From the campfire where people tell stories about victorious battles in order to raise everyone's fighting spirit or the porch where people share the wonder of seeing shooting stars while someone can be overheard singing the Bangles. A whole life so lonely, and then we come together and ease the pain. Am I only dreaming? Or is this burning an eternal flame?

Do you feel the same?

Forever yours, Vilja

PS

This letter is an assemblage of words and situations created by friends and comrades around the world. Despite having one writer, it is a collaboration of many, not only because of the borrowed words, but due to all the shared magic and intense discussions. As you already should know, I love all of you very much!

❈ ❈ ❈

Vilja Saarinen writes from Helsinki, although she would love to be with you, wherever you are and wherever there is even a tiny spark. Vilja finds it important to appreciate and celebrate our big and small victories throughout history, and never forget the beauty of our resistance. If you feel the same, feel free to write to her at viljasaarinen@protonmail.com.

## IF YOU LIKED THIS BOOK, SEE MILSTEIN'S PREVIOUS TITLES, ALL LABORS OF LOVE:

*Anarchism and Its Aspirations*, by Cindy Milstein (AK Press, 2010)

*Paths toward Utopia: Graphic Explorations of Everyday Anarchism*, by Cindy Milstein and Erik Ruin (PM Press, 2012)

*Taking Sides: Revolutionary Solidarity and the Poverty of Liberalism*, edited by Cindy Milstein (AK Press, 2015)

*Rebellious Mourning: The Collective Work of Grief*, edited by Cindy Milstein (AK Press, 2017)

*Deciding for Ourselves: The Promise of Direct Democracy*, edited by Cindy Milstein (AK Press, 2020)

*There Is Nothing So Whole as a Broken Heart: Mending the World as Jewish Anarchists*, edited by Cindy Milstein (AK Press, 2021)

*Try Anarchism for Life: The Beauty of Our Circle*, by Cindy Barukh Milstein (Strangers in a Tangled Wilderness, 2022)